DENTISTRY
SHAKEN AND STIRRED

Health and Controversy in Your Mouth

CINDY MAY GROSSMANN, R.D.H.

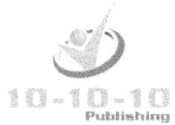

Dentistry Shaken & Stirred: Health and Controversy in Your Mouth

www.dentistryshakenandstirred.com

Copyright © 2020 Cindy Grossmann

ISBN: 979-8558914818

All rights reserved. No portion of this book may be reproduced mechanically, electronically, or by any other means, including photocopying, without permission of the publisher or author except in the case of brief quotations embodied in critical articles and reviews. It is illegal to copy this book, post it to a website, or distribute it by any other means without permission from the publisher or author.

Limits of Liability and Disclaimer of Warranty

The author and publisher shall not be liable for your misuse of the enclosed material. This book is strictly for informational and educational purposes only.

Warning – Disclaimer

The purpose of this book is to educate and entertain. The author and/or publisher do not guarantee that anyone following these techniques, suggestions, tips, ideas, or strategies will become successful. The author and/or publisher shall have neither liability nor responsibility to anyone with respect to any loss or damage caused, or alleged to be caused, directly or indirectly by the information contained in this book.

Medical Disclaimer

The medical or health information in this book is provided as an information resource only, and is not to be used or relied on for any diagnostic or treatment purposes. This information is not intended to be patient education, does not create any patient-physician relationship, and should not be used as a substitute for professional diagnosis and treatment.

Publisher
10-10-10 Publishing
Markham, ON Canada

Printed in the United States of America

Created for the photo on the cover – Dan Anderson, "Eastern State Penitentiary Chair" – Flickr, 20 August 2015 – www.flickr.com/photos/stonebridgedapper/20858584420

Dedicated to Dan Grossmann (1962-2011) - An entrepreneur who never quit. Thank you for showing me entrepreneurship years before I was ready. Thank you for supporting me in all my careers through the years. One day we will meet again.

CONTENTS

ACKNOWLEDGEMENTS ix

INTRODUCTION 1

1. BE THE ALTERNATIVE 5
   Spirituality 7
   Traditional Chinese Medicine (TCM) 9
   Emotional Freedom Technique (EFT) 10
   Palmistry 11
   Reflexology 12
   Hand Reflexology 13
   Yoga 14
   Chakras 14

2. MORE ALTERNATIVELY SPEAKING 19
   Reiki 21
   Homeopathy 22
   Platelet Rich Plasma (PRP) 23
   Crystals and Healing Stones 23
   Hirudotherapy 24
   Essential Oils 25
   Tongue Diagnosis 26
   Ayurveda 29
   Aromatherapy 31

3. WHAT'S EATING YOU? 33
   Types of Teeth 35
   Wisdom Teeth 38
   Tonsils 39
   Lip Lifts 40
   Botox 42
   Nightguards 44
   What You Should Know About Lipstick 46

4. DOES MILK DO A BODY GOOD? 49
   What is in Our Milk? 51
   The Downsides of Drinking Cow's Milk 55
   Important Dates in Milk History 57

5. LET'S GET TO THE ROOT OF IT 67
   Root Canal Therapy 69
   Are Root Canals Necessary? 73
   Root Canals in Primary Teeth 77
   Nitrous Oxide 79

6. THE 60 SECOND TREATMENT 83
   Fluoride 85
   Different Types of Fluoride 86
   Can Fluoride be Harmful to You? 87

7. MERCURY RISING 101
   Amalgam Restorations 103
   Diseases Linked to Mercury 106
   Precautions and Removal Process of Mercury Fillings 110

8. ONE OF THESE THINGS JUST DOESN'T BELONG 115
   Why is that in Your Mouth? 117
   Ingredients in Toothpaste 119
   Cavitations 122
   Let's Keep it Clean 123

9. IT'S A DOG'S LIFE 131
   Animals and Their Mouths 134
   Dental Care for Your Animal 140
   Your Pet's Tongue 142
   What to Avoid Giving Your Dog 143

10. BUT WAIT THERE'S MORE 145
    Fun Facts 147

ACKNOWLEDGEMENTS

To my children, **Drew Grossmann and Michael Grossmann** – I am proud of all your accomplishments and will continue to support them. I am so proud to have you both as my sons! Thank you for your supporting me and wanting me to be happy. And thank you for always taking such great care of your teeth!

Drew – I am so proud of your business building. You're an amazing public speaker and your knowledge is endless. I love learning from you. I am very excited for all the great things that will come to you. And I am so proud and impressed with all your hard work.

Mike – I am so proud of all your hard work as well. You are such a great actor and model, and you have such range of character. Your charm and charisma will certainly take you very far and I can't wait to be there to watch! I have seen you accomplish great things that you set your mind to!

Buddy – You are the reason they say dogs are man's best friend. I couldn't ask for a better BFF.

Mel May – My dad, thank you for asking me about this book and encouraging me all the time. And for listening to what I had to say.

Harriet Dank and Bob Dank – My mom and stepfather thank you for supporting me, asking about my book all the time and questioning what I was doing.

My brothers, Arnold May and Bernie May – Thank you for keeping up with what I am doing and asking me questions.

Sami, Michele, Dan and Logan T – Thank you for your friendship and for taking such great care of Buddy! You are the best!

Olivia C – Thank you for the overnights you spent with Buddy so I could take my courses. Thank you for all the amazing photos and long walks with him as well!

Dr Alex C, thank you for the cover photo inspiration. I am grateful we remained friends after I inspected your office years ago. Thank you for certifying me to teach CPR and encouraging me to write and teach CEU courses.

Raymond A – Thank you for publishing this book so others can learn what they may not know. I appreciate you teaching me 10-10-10 so that I could write to teach others. Thank you for sharing Mulberry Hill with me as well. And thank you for the Monthly Mentor program.

Danielle P – My go-to person at Raymond Aaron Group, you are an amazing friend. Thank you for all your help!

Liz V – Thank you for all the back and forth emails keeping up with me and the book changes!

Lisa B – Thank you for taking your time and proofreading this!

Sam C – Thank you for all you help in getting my podcast up and running. Your help and all of your honesty are greatly appreciated. You are a great coach and your knowledge is priceless!

Acknowledgements

Mark Y – Thank you beyond words! Your availability and your love are much appreciated always!

Cheryl W – Thank you for being an amazing teacher, friend and worker!

Dee Dee S – From coach to friend thank you for all your input!

My SRA friends and PTI friends – I am grateful to you and love seeing everyone's successes!

Dr. Daniel W – Being in the dental field, I couldn't understand why as a pediatrician, you were against fluoride. But I understand years later. Thank you for your honesty back then.

Chevelle C – My first dental patient. I forgot to give you a fluoride treatment. Perhaps it was not a mistake and subconsciously I knew something more.

Chrissy K – Thank you for teaching me what I rolled my eyes at then and cannot unsee now!

My Yoga teachers – Thank you for the time in the hot room!

Jess A – I love your words "Do it now before it's too late and you can't tie your shoes."

Chrissy D – "Self Care is Your Divine Responsibility." Thank you for the reminder always!

Paul L – My yoga form would not be what it is without your teachings. I am constantly learning!

David L – You are an amazing Latin and Ballroom teacher! I love all our crazy routines!

Jumin E. K – Eternally grateful on so many levels. You challenge and motivate me!

Jim Mc C – Your 10-year friendship, kindness and generosity to me and my boys is priceless!

Salvatore B – Thank you for your friendship!

Debbie B – I am so glad we met on the commercial set years ago and stayed great friends!

Joe O and OK Sports Marketing – Thank you for the marketing ideas and long-time friendship.

Jesus R – From NYC to Cali, thank you for your friendship and daily encouragement!

Robert T – I am so glad we got to work together on TV and movie sets and remained friends!

Dan D – Thank you for always supporting me and keeping me up to date on new dance steps!

Toni A – Thanks for keeping up on all I have done over the years and giving me input. Thank you also to Frank and Ricky for their love and support!

Tammy B And Karen B – My longtime RDH friends. I am glad we are still close!

Len V – Thank you for all the articles! And for your encouragement!

Dawn R – Thank you for the most amazing modeling photos!

Patti D – Always love discussing the universe with you!

Acknowledgements

Jawanda J – Thank you for your support!

Vu T – Your knowledge has helped me tremendously! I appreciate all your input!

Michele R. – I am so glad we are friends!

American Express – I am indebted to you, no pun intended. Without you I could not have gotten where I am!

To the Universe – Thank you for allowing the most amazing wonderful things and people to manifest into my life in ways I could never have imagined!

All of my "Brilliant Smiles by Cindy" clients – Thank you for trusting me to make your smiles whiter and brighter!

To everyone on social media who doesn't know me personally but trusts me enough to ask me questions – Thank you!!!

You the reader – Thank you for taking your time to read this. I hope you pick up some information you did not know before!

INTRODUCTION

"You can't see what you don't know and you can't know what you don't see but once you know you can't unknow and once you see you can't unsee."

—Cindy

Health…. Dentistry…. Deception. Dental treatment … it's meant to correct your smile, enhance your smile and bring health to your smile … and health to your body… but at what cost? What lies behind the mask of dentistry? Dental care should be for life… but is some treatment, or lack thereof, shortening yours?

Did you know that according to some studies 98% of women with breast cancer have had a root canal on that side of their mouth? Did you know that certain lipstick shades can make your teeth appear different shades? Did you know that people, as well as animals, are more attracted to happy rather than sad people? Did you know that magnesium helps build strong bones even more importantly than calcium?

What is better, a silver (mercury) filling or a white (composite) filling? Do you need to get your wisdom teeth out? Is fluoride the best thing to prevent a cavity or is fluoride a neurotoxin? Where did the term Mad Hatter Disease come from? Why are there warning labels on toothpaste? Did you know three tablespoons of chia seeds have more than double the calcium of a glass of milk (631 mg vs 300 mg)? One and a half cups of chickpeas has a little more calcium than a glass of milk (315mg vs 300 mg). And three quarters of a cup of almonds beats the calcium in milk as well (320 mg vs 300 mg).

Did you know that besides eyes, a smile is the first thing to be noticed? It has been proven that people who smile are more successful. What is the first thing you think of in the morning? Is it what clothes you will wear? What shoes? What lipstick? Or if you will smile? It is said that a smile is the universal language of kindness, and that when you smile, the whole world smiles with you. Your smile is your business card and it is more than merely 17 muscles that make this happen.

We start to smile before we are even born, as evidenced on 4-D ultrasounds. Once we are 6-8 weeks old, we smile with definitive intention. This is also about the time babies vision expands and they look at people's faces with purpose. Since smiles are known to be contagious, you can't help but smile around a baby. Children smile approximately 400 times a day, yet adults smile approximately 20 times per day. Happy adults smile 40-50 times per day.

There are 19 different types of smiles with the most natural one is known as the Duchenne smile. In this smile the corners of your lips turn up and your cheeks are raised. Also crow's feet are formed by your eyes in a Duchenne smile. It is also said this type of smile is genuine and can't be faked. It has been shown that 48 percent of people have untagged themselves from Facebook because they did not like their smile. 61 percent of people say they are attracted to someone solely because of their smile. On average women smile 62 times a day while on average men smile only 8 times per day. It is good to know that smiling does not cause smile lines but smiling does make you appear on average 2 years younger! Your face can make over 5000 expressions and has only 43 muscles.

Introduction

Fifty percent of people say they get put into a better mood once a stranger smiles at them. And almost 100% of people believe smiling makes them feel better. Smiling can even boost your immune system. Your smile projects how you feel inside, and can show on the outside. Your energy can shift just by smiling.

It is not only humans that are attracted by a smile. Research has shown that animals gravitate to happy people and photos of people who are smiling.

What goes into the making of a happy smile? A healthy smile both inside and out?

This book is not intended to give or promote medical and or dental treatment or advice. Consult your dental or medical provider for questions and advice on treatment. This book is not a substitute for medical and or dental advice and/or treatment.

This book is based on research and facts, a lot of which I was not taught in Dental Hygiene school or in continuing education courses. I want to share my knowledge so that you can make the right decisions for yourself and know it is okay to ask questions and be your own advocate. No one knows what is best for you, except you. Nothing in here is a substitute for professional advice and nothing in here is telling you what to do.

This book could teach you the basics on how to brush, floss and rinse, but I wanted to bring something more to light. Some things that your dental professionals may not tell you and they may not even know. So much of your health can be determined just by taking a look inside your smile (no pun intended).

CHAPTER 1
BE THE ALTERNATIVE

SPIRITUALITY

There is a lot of confusion when it comes to spirituality because there is no single meaning to the term spirituality in today's world. Spirituality was first noted in the 5th century and had a religious background, then the meaning changed in the 11th century. During the 19th and 20th centuries the concept of spirituality separated from religiousness.

Here are two modern-day experts' definitions of the word spirituality:

Christina Puchalski, MD, Director of the George Washington Institute for Spirituality and Health, says that "spirituality is the aspect of humanity that refers to the way individuals seek and express meaning and purpose, and the way they experience their connectedness to the moment, to self, to others, to nature, and to the significant or sacred."

Mario Beauregard and Denyse O'Leary are researchers and the authors of *The Spiritual Brain* and they say spirituality is "any experience that is thought to bring the experiencer into contact with the divine. In other words, not just any experience that feels meaningful."

Although spirituality and religion are not the same thing, they do have some overlapping qualities.

People that are spiritual believe that tooth issues are associated with mental wellbeing and each tooth has a specific thought or feeling to bring out symptoms.

Dr Michael Caffin is a well-known French oral surgeon and came up with the following link with regard to each specific tooth. The teeth mentioned below are in the permanent dentition of one's mouth.

Teeth numbers 1-8 (upper right quadrant of your mouth which would include 8 teeth if all are present) are connected to wanting to express yourself. Any issues occurring in these teeth signify a difficulty in feeling safe in the outside world. Teeth numbers 9-16 (the 8 teeth making up the upper left quadrant of your mouth) are associated with wanting to project what you are feeling inside. An issue in this quadrant of the mouth is indicative of a hard time fulfilling your want to just be.

Teeth numbers 17-24 (lower left quadrant of 8 teeth) are linked to the awareness of self inner vulnerabilities. Problems with teeth in this quadrant show an absence of emotional identification amongst family.

Teeth numbers 25-32 (the lower right quadrant of 8 teeth) are attached to having things such as work become concrete. Concerns with these teeth are linked to problems with solidifying plans and things.

Not everyone has wisdom teeth (teeth numbers 1,16,17 and 32), but these tend to be the teeth causing the most problems. Spiritual meaning of pain includes judging and criticizing yourself.

Tooth decay in spirituality is said to mean the belief of criticism of oneself. It is also linked to extremely low self-esteem, withholding approval and feeling unappreciated.

It is said that one side of your body represents the feminine side and one side the masculine. The feminine side is where we pull in and the masculine side of the body is where we voice out. In spirituality, the relationship with your father is controlled on the right side of your body. That being said, any unresolved issues with your father would show on this side of your mouth. The left side represents mother relationship and issues.

There are many charts that can be assessed which show individual characteristics of teeth and what modalities in your personal life affect them in order for you to recognize them.

TRADITIONAL CHINESE MEDICINE (TCM)

There are no records dating back prior to the second century BC when it comes to medical practicing techniques, but this is when Traditional Chinese Medicine (TCM) is said to have started. TCM includes such treatments as acupuncture, diet, herbs, exercise and moxibustion. In TCM, it is said that Kidney Qi (pronounced 'chee') is directly related to the health of teeth and bones. Qi is what keeps a person in balance, physically, mentally, emotionally, and spiritually. Energy flow is said to run through the full body and must remain flowing or health issues arise. Meridians are the map of the flow of QI or energy in the body. Meridians are also referred to as acupuncture points. Acupuncture is the opening of specific meridians for a harmonious energy (Qi) flow. Acupuncture uses thin needles which are inserted in specific body points depending on the condition it is treating in the session. The needles are left in for 5 - 30 minutes, and the treatment is usually painless. To date only four acupuncture points are known in the mouth; however, there are multiple points on one's body which correspond to the mouth and oral health issues.

Acupuncture has been known to help alleviate oral issues such as dry mouth, (xerostomia), toothache, periodontal disease and dental anxiety, just to name a few. Every person has 12 main meridians, which relate to organs and glands. In TCM the words teeth and bones are synonymous. A strong Kidney Qi translates to a healthy mouth. In TCM all teeth are on a specific meridian in the body. Also, on this meridian is an organ in direct correlation to each tooth. The meridian chart has a detailed listing for each tooth which includes the organs, joints, vertebrae, endocrine systems and muscles as they connect to each tooth individually. Not all meridian charts are exactly the same.

In Western Medicine the human body is like a machine. Broken parts are removed or if possible they are fixed. In Chinese Medicine the body is thought of as a garden. Soil is checked when the leaves are not at their peak. Chinese medicine explores the root of the problem rather than just addressing the specific problem.

EMOTIONAL FREEDOM TECHNIQUE (EFT)

Emotional Freedom Technique (EFT) was discovered by Gary Craig in the 1900s. It is known as EFT or EFT tapping, and is used for both physical and emotional distress. It has been shown that when you tap near a specific point on a meridian you alleviate physical issues and you also feel better. EFT is a system in which it is believed all problems stem from emotions and once the emotion is eliminated or at least reduced, the physical ailment follows in relief.

The mechanics of how tapping works is pretty simple. Calming signals are sent to the stress center of the brain, which releases negative emotions and thoughts once an area is "tapped." EFT is a simple and pain-free, drug-free system which can be learned easily and done on your own. EFT follows the principle that, when the body's energy system flows freely, negative emotions are released. Acupuncture was put in place for physical ailments and EFT tapping is sometimes referred to as "emotional acupuncture" or "energy psychology."

There are numerous success stories of using EFT for tooth grinding, pain and dental fear. It is important to note that when using EFT, it is not required or even recommended to pull up emotional trauma from the past in order to relive it. EFT has shown promising results in the dental field. It has been said that EFT also helps with toothaches, and sore swollen gums. This type of self-treatment can be done either sitting, standing or lying down. Over 100 studies have proven EFT to be effective, including a study done at Harvard.

PALMISTRY

The exact origin of Palmistry or palm reading is not known but is believed to have originated in India. It is also been said that the left hand is what you are given, and the right hand is what you do or do not do with what you've been given. It has been found that events in your life can change the lines on your palms and/or fingers. It is also believed that your dominant hand would see the most changes and is the hand to be read. Tooth and gum issues can be located on the palm by looking at the "heart line." The heart line runs across the palm starting at either your first or middle finger. This line ends by your pinky. Also determined by markings on the heart line is a timing of life events early years, adulthood and senior years.

There are many variations which can be seen in all your palm lines. These include but are not limited to circles, islands, crosses, dots, curves, broken and deep-set lines. It has been said that, if your heart line has vertical lines which cross it under your middle fingers, it is an indication of problems with your teeth and your gums.

REFLEXOLOGY

The origin of reflexology is not clearly known. It is said to have been used in China as well as in Egypt in approximately the year 2330 BC. Reflexology comes from the word "reflux," meaning "an involuntary or instinctive movement in response to a stimulus." Reflexology is massaging specific points on the feet, hands and or head to treat illness and relieve stress. There are specific points on all three of these areas which link to specific body parts, and will alleviate pain and or tension in the corresponding body parts when they are activated

Chinese reflexology to help with your teeth is on the top part of your toes. The toes on your right foot are for teeth on the left side of your mouth and the toes on your left foot are for teeth on the right side of your mouth. The points to stimulate are above and below the knuckle on your toes. Massaging above the knuckle will deal with your upper teeth, hence massaging below the toe knuckle will alleviate pain from lower teeth. There is also a tooth reflexology chart in which each tooth represents one or more organs.

The four wisdom teeth (numbers 1,16,17,32) are related to the heart and small intestine. The first and second molars on the right side of the mouth and both upper and lower arches (numbers 2,3,30,31) represent stomach pancreas, and thyroid. The first and second molars on the left , both upper and lower arches (numbers 14,15,18,19), represent stomach, spleen, and thyroid. All eight premolars (numbers 4,5,12,13,20,21,28,29) represent lungs and colon. All four canines (numbers 6,11,22,27) represent liver and gallbladder. The four lateral incisors (numbers 7,10,23,26) along with the four central incisors (numbers 8,9,24,25) represent kidney, bladder, prostate, and uterus.

As you can see, everything is uniform and equal on both sides, except the first and second molars on the right side, which are pancreas-related whereas the first and second molars on the left side are spleen-related. A baby has feet that are divided into six zones. Zone number one is the toes, and this is where head and teeth issues are to be massaged. You will be able to tell if you are healing, as the sensitivity level when you massage points on your feet is less, as is the energy to that part of the body. When using reflexology to heal an issue on the left side of your body, you'd massage the reflexology point on the right foot and vice versa. Reflexology has been known to help with headaches, toothaches, and speeding up healing from dental work, just to name a few.

HAND REFLEXOLOGY

Hand reflexology got its beginnings at the same time as foot reflexology did. The hands have points which also mirror body parts. Hand reflexology is another method that when used by yourself is sometimes easier. Each one of your hands has sixteen points that relate to your teeth. The hand used is the one on the same side of your body as the tooth issue. In each quadrant of your mouth there are eight teeth and they are represented by a certain finger.

Your index finger holds clues to teeth numbers 1 and 2 (wisdom tooth and second molar). Middle finger is teeth 3 and 4 (first molar and second premolar). Ring finger is numbers 5 and 6 (first premolar and canine), followed by your pinky for teeth numbers 7 and 8 (lateral incisor and central incisor). Follow this pattern for the other three quadrants. Hand reflexology uses the top knuckle (the one closest to your fingernails on each finger. Massaging above this knuckle is for upper teeth while right below the knuckle is for lower teeth.

The exact point to massage or hold is on the corners of the knuckle. You count the tooth number the same way on toe points to identify the area for specific tooth numbers. Hand reflexology has been shown to help relieve a toothache, speed healing of a dental abscess and to help babies with teething pain, just to name a few.

YOGA

Yoga has been around for over 5000 years and has its beginning in Northern India. The word yoga has its origin from the Sanskrit word "Yuj," which is translated as unite or join. Yoga joins to the body and the mind by breathing through postures. Yoga has been shown to be beneficial to dental health in several ways. Yoga helps with posture, and proper posture can keep your jaw aligned properly.

Yoga has also been shown to increase the flow of saliva. Saliva is needed to help break food down when chewing, and also in the prevention of dry mouth syndrome. Yoga also helps reduce anxiety and migraines. Some studies show using yoga can help with toothaches as well. By doing yoga, you are reducing your stress level, and stress is a contributing factor in clenching or grinding your teeth, Also, by reducing stress levels, you are reducing your chances of gum inflammation.

CHAKRAS

The "Chakra" system has its origin in India sometime between 1500 and 500 BC. The word chakra is defined as a wheel, as in a wheel of energy throughout your body. There are seven main chakras throughout the body.

The goal is to keep these wheels of energy open as they determine our psychological, emotional and spiritual states. These chakras are also comprised of nerves and organs. Not only is it believed that each tooth is associated with meridians in your body, but teeth are also associated with emotions, organs and chakras.

The first chakra is the "Root Chakra" and is located at the base of the spine. The second chakra is the "Sacral Chakra," just below the navel. The third chakra is the "Solar Plexus Chakra" and is located in your stomach area. The fourth chakra is the "Heart Chakra," located in the center your chest. The fifth Chakra is the "Throat Chakra," located at the base of your throat. The sixth chakra is the "Third Eye Chakra," and is located on your forehead, between your eyes and above them. The seventh chakra is the "Crown Chakra," and is located on the top of your head. Chakras one, two and three are dealing with matter, chakras five, six and seven deal with spirit, and the fourth chakra is the connection between the two. The fifth chakra is the chakra associated with the jaw, tongue and mouth. When your fifth chakra is blocked it can manifest itself as a sore throat, a thyroid problem, tension headaches or neck and shoulder pain.

The following is a reference of some key emotions, meridians or organs and chakras believed to be associated with each tooth. Note these are all permanent teeth being referenced and also note this is just a few points listed. Teeth numbers 1,16,17 and 32 are wisdom teeth, also known as third molars and they are not always present in the mouth.

Here are some specifics on each tooth:

Tooth #1 (UR third molar) loneliness or trapped / endocrine and/or small intestine / throat, heart, solar plexus, sacral, root chakras

Tooth #2 (UR second molar) anxiety / stomach and/or right breast / throat, heart, solar plexus, sacral, root chakras

Tooth #3 (UR first molar) anxiety or low self- esteem / right breast and/or stomach / throat, heart, solar plexus, sacral, root chakras

Tooth #4 (UR second premolar) control fear or sadness / large intestines or lungs / throat, heart, solar plexus chakras

Tooth #5 (UR first premolar) control fear or sadness / large intestines or lungs / throat, heart, solar plexus chakras

Tooth #6 (UR canine) anger or resentment / liver or gall bladder / throat, solar plexus chakras

Tooth #7 (UR lateral incisor) fatigue or fear or guilt / kidney or bladder / throat, solar plexus, sacral, root chakras

Tooth #8 (UR central incisor) fatigue or fear or guilt / kidney or bladder / throat, solar plexus, sacral, root chakras

Tooth #9 (UL central incisor) fatigue or fear or guilt / kidney or bladder / throat, solar plexus, sacral, root chakras

Tooth #10 (UL lateral incisor) fatigue or fear or guilt / kidney or bladder / throat, solar plexus sacral, root chakras

Tooth #11 (UL canine) anger or manipulation / liver or gall bladder / throat, solar plexus chakras

Tooth #12 (UL first premolar) control fear or sadness / large intestine or lungs / throat, heart, solar plexus chakras

Tooth #13 (UL second premolar) control fear or sadness / large intestine or lungs / heart, solar plexus chakras

Tooth #14 (UL first molar) anxiety or low self-esteem / stomach or left breast / throat, solar plexus, sacral, root chakras

Tooth #15 (UL second molar) anxiety or low self-esteem / stomach or left breast / throat, solar plexus, sacral, root chakras

Tooth #16 (UL third molar) loneliness or trapped / endocrine or small intestine / throat, heart, solar plexus, sacral, root chakras

Tooth #17 (LL third molar) loneliness or trapped / endocrine or small intestine / throat, heart, solar plexus, sacral, root chakras

Tooth #18 (LL second molar). control fear or sadness / large intestine or lungs, throat, heart, solar plexus chakras

Tooth #19 (LL first molar) control fear or sadness / large intestine or lungs / throat, heart, solar plexus chakras

Tooth #20 (LL second premolar) anxiety or low self-esteem / stomach or left breast / solar plexus, sacral, root chakras

Tooth #21 (LL first premolar). anxiety or low self-esteem, stomach or left breast / throat, heart, solar plexus, sacral, root chakras

Tooth #22 (LL canine). anger or resentment / liver or gall bladder / throat, solar plexus chakras

Tooth #23 (LL lateral incisor) fear or guilt / kidney or bladder / throat, solar plexus, sacral, root chakras

Tooth #24 (LL central incisor) fear or guilt / kidney or bladder / throat, solar plexus, sacral, root chakras

Tooth #25 (LR central incisor) fear or guilt / kidney or bladder / throat, solar plexus, sacral, root chakras

Tooth #26 (LR lateral incisor). fear or guilt / kidney or bladder/ throat, solar plexus, sacral, root chakras

Tooth #27 (LR canine). anger or resentment / liver or gall bladder / throat, solar plexus chakras

Tooth #28 (LR first premolar). anxiety or low self-esteem/ right breast or stomach/ throat, heart, solar plexus, sacral, root chakras

Tooth #29 (LR second premolar). anxiety or low self-esteem/ right breast or stomach/ throat, heart, solar plexus, sacral, root chakras

Tooth #30 (LR first molar) control fear or sadness / large intestine or lungs/ throat, heart, solar- chakras

Tooth #31 (LR second molar) control fear or sadness/ large intestine or lungs / throat, heart, solar plexus chakras

Tooth #32 (LR third molar). Loneliness or unloved / endocrine or small intestine/ throat, heart, solar plexus, sacral, root chakras

CHAPTER 2
MORE ALTERNATIVELY SPEAKING

REIKI

Reiki was founded by Dr. Mikao Usui, who was born in 1865, and in 1922 opened his first Reiki school and clinic in Japan. Reiki is another form of energy healing, and reiki practitioners use chakras for points of reference in their healings. Reiki can be done with the practitioner touching the patient lightly or even not touching the patient at all. Healing energy is transferred from the practitioner's palms to the patient and the body responds by healing naturally. Reiki is used for both emotional and physical healing. The word Reiki as defined in IARP.org comes from two Japanese words, "Rei," defined as "Universal Life","Ki," meaning "Energy."

Reiki is simple and pain-free, and can treat the whole body. It also can work in conjunction with other treatments the patient is receiving as there are no side effects or contraindications. Reiki is not a religion as there is nothing which you must believe in order to learn reiki. One must receive an "attunement" by a reiki master in order to receive the ability to use this. By a reiki practitioner placing his or her palms on the jaw, throat and the organs associated with your teeth, it will promote healing. Remember, if you do not want the practitioner to touch you, they can hold their hands close to your body.

Reiki practitioners can help to heal any of the seven blocked chakras as well. An average reiki session is 60 minutes. You will be fully clothed, and will lie on your back, or if you prefer, you may be semi-reclined in a chair during your session. Reiki has been said to be helpful with toothache, gum disease and headaches, to name a few.

HOMEOPATHY

Homeopathy is based on the principle of "like cures like." Samuel Hahnemann is the founder of homeopathy in 1796, basing the system on the claim a small amount of the symptom you are experiencing is given to trigger the body heal itself. Homeopathic remedies are from plants, minerals or animals. An easy example to understand the premise of homeopathy is as follows. Onions cause eyes to water and turn red. Hence when eyes are watery and red due to allergies the onion remedy (Allium Cepa) is given, Another example is itching caused by poison ivy is treated with a remedy (Rhus Tox) made from poison ivy.

These products are sold as dissolvable tablets, creams, ointments and pellets. Pellets are sold in different strengths such as 6C, 6X, 30C, 200C. Every pellet, no matter the strength or the remedy, looks and tastes the same. The difference in the strength is determined by its dilution power. Pellets are placed under the tongue to dissolve or they can be diluted in water and the water is shaken before consuming. This also makes a remedy stronger. It is recommended to not eat or drink thirty minutes prior to taking homeopathic remedies. Another important principle in homeopathy is that it is the symptom that is treated, not the disease. There can be multiple people with the same dental issues and it is possible for them to be given a different remedy or set of remedies. It is also possible, once symptoms subside or change, for your remedy to be changed or altered. In order to become a homeopathic practitioner, you must attend medical training and get a license. Homeopaths are also required to have thirty hours of continuing education every three years.

Homeopathy has shown to be helpful with dental phobia, toothache, healing and to name a few. Some helpful remedies for common dental ailments include, Belladonna for toothache and for grinding. Natrum muriaticum is said to help fever blisters, cold sores, and cracking in the corners of the mouth. Arsenicum album is for bleeding gums and pulp issues. Chamomile and Calcarea Carbonica are believed to help toothaches. Aconite is said to be useful in panic or fear incidences. Homeopathy is a simple, effective, and inexpensive treatment for many dental issues and is available over the counter.

PLATELET RICH PLASMA (PRP)

PRP is a relatively new adjunct in dentistry. Platelet Rich Plasma, as it is also known, uses your own blood. After drawing blood it is spun in a centrifuge to remove the red blood cells. The platelets are then re-injected into specific targeted area(s) of your body for regeneration and growth and/or healing. PRP is being used to help in oral surgery with healing wounds and regenerating bone. PRP was given its own CPT code on July 1, 2010. A CPT code is the code which is used on an insurance claim for reimbursement of fees. PRP benefits healing by covering a wound and minimizing the possibility of infection. Tissues also heal faster when PRP is incorporated into treatment. Platelets in the blood are what heal the wounds, and rejection is a non-issue since it is your own blood. The first time PRP was used in surgery was 1987.

CRYSTALS AND HEALING STONES

It is a known fact that everything is energy. Even things that are solid are made up of energy. Your body is made up of energy and so are stones or crystals, although none of this is visible to the naked eye. When a crystal is placed on your body, the energy is transformed and vibrates in accordance to the specific property of said crystal. Different crystals are meant for different things as their energies are different. Crystals are like magnets, in that they can attract and remove negative energies from your body.

Crystals can be worn, placed directly on specific body parts, or even just kept close by while you sleep, in order to work their magic. Malachite and Aquamarine are the stones to use for pain relief. Amber is the stone to use to help teething pain in children. If you need a stone for facial pain, you would choose Beryl or you would want to hold a Fluorite stone. Crystals go back a long time in history for healing usage. People use healing crystals to help with toothache, tooth decay, bad breath and for preventative measures, to name a few.

HIRUDOTHERAPY

You may not have heard of Hiruotherapy, but you have probably heard of leeches and leech therapy or healing. Leech therapy is also known as Hirudotherapy and dates back to the Egyptians. Over the centuries it has been used worldwide in the treatment of illnesses. Medicinal leeches were cleared by the FDA for usage on June 28, 2004 and medicinal leeches were also deemed synonymous with the definition of a medical device. Medicinal leeches are being used in today's medicine for treatment of gum disease amongst other oral issues.

Leeches work by first releasing anesthesia to you while they are eating your blood. Next is the vasodilator, this gets the blood to flow where the leech bite is and makes the leech suck more blood. Next the anticoagulant keeps your blood from clotting. Finally the platelets are kept from sticking together by platelet aggregation. Once a leech is used for healing, it cannot be used on another person or sent back into wild, so it is killed. Hirudotherapy has shown promise for dentistry as it reduces inflammation and inhibits bacteria from continuing to grow.

ESSENTIAL OILS

Egyptians usually get credited for the beginning of the usage of essential oils, around the time of 3000-2500 BC. However, it seems oils were being used in China and India as well. Essential oils come from plants and evaporate easily at a normal temperature (they are known as volatile). These oils have the essence of the plant they are derived from and thus called "essential." Since essential oils come from nature it is impossible to have a patent on them. (Essential oils are not even oils since they do not contain any fatty acids.)

Essential oils are either diffused and inhaled, or massaged onto the skin using a carrier oil. Massaging oils into your skin, especially on the bottom of your feet, can make them take effect in less than 1/2 hour. It is said that oils stimulate your sense of smell and have medicinal effects on the body. Studies show that you can raise your vibration and body frequency by using essential oils.

To determine the frequency of one's body, a biofeedback machine would be used. These machines work by measuring brain waves and/or skin temperature. The average healthy human has a 62-72 MHz (megahertz). Rose oil is said to have the highest frequency, measuring 320 MHz. The MHz of some other common essential oils are: lavender 118 MHz and frankincense 147 MHz. By diffusing oils or using them topically, you are getting the benefits of these high frequencies. You can also raise your frequency by positive thinking (just as you can lower your frequency by negative thinking).

Essential oils are very concentrated and are best kept in dark glass bottles. They should be stored in a cool and dry place in order to prolong shelf life. When essential oils come in contact with the skin, results can take effect in as little twenty minutes. Essential oils have been shown to improve confidence, lift spirits, and boost your immune system. In regards to dentistry they have been shown to increase circulation, reduce anxiety, help with toothaches and reduce headaches, to name a few. Studies have been shown that using essential oils for wound dressing results in better healing. Anti-plaque mouth rinses made with essential oils have also been shown to work and may not cause staining of teeth.

TONGUE DIAGNOSIS

Your tongue is the only muscle which you can see. The pink flesh of your tongue is called mucosa. The rough texture is due to papillae, which are the tiny bumps you see covering your tongue. There are five types of taste buds (and thousands of them on your tongue) and these taste buds cover the papillae. These five taste buds include sweet, sour, bitter, salty and umami. Umami is responsible for the sensation you get when tasting glutamate. The tongue is an important muscle as it is necessary for speech, eating and swallowing.

Underneath your tongue is a muscle called the frenum, which anchors the tongue to the floor of the mouth. There are two other frenum in front of your mouth. They are the attachments your lip has to your gums. Sometimes one or all of these frenums need to be cut to allow for proper motion of the tongue, or because the frenum is causing the gum to recede and needs to be released. Geographic tongue shows up in 2-3 % of people. The etiology is unknown and it is usually benign with no problems. It occurs on top of the tongue (dorsal) and is characterized by areas that look like a map. The reddened smooth areas are caused by loss of papillae. These areas do move from time to time. There is no protocol to treat this condition and it does not cause pain.

In Chinese medicine the tongue is always looked at and analyzed for diagnosis. In TCM it is believed the tongue can show the health of the liver, lung, spleen, heart and kidney. There are ten types of tongues in TCM. Using the tongue as a diagnostic tool dates back to the times before X-rays and other imaging tools were available. It is still a widely used tool to determine full body health.

Here are the 10 types of tongue diagnoses:

1. "Normal" tongue is a pink or light red colored tongue.
2. "Qi Deficiency" tongue is a pale tongue having a few red spots and a thin white coating. People exhibiting "Qi Deficiency" have symptoms such as fatigue and poor appetite. They also tend to overthink and worry.
3. "Heat" tongue is red with a thin yellow coating. These people feel hot thirsty and constipated. They sweat easily and are irritable. They may also have skin issues.
4. "Damp Retention" tongue is a swollen tongue with a white greasy coating. Symptoms are bloating, lethargy and fullness in chest and abdomen.
5. "Blood Stasis" tongue is a purple colored tongue with black spots on it. Symptoms include varicose veins, painful legs, headaches and non-lustrous skin.
6. "Qi Stagnation" tongue is a tongue with a red tip. These people are in an unstable emotional state and have a tendency to be depressed.

7. "Damp Heat" tongue is a tongue which is red with a greasy yellow coating. Symptoms include skin issues, UTI, clamminess and anger.

8. "Yang Deficiency" tongue is a pale and swollen tongue with a thick white coating. Symptoms include back pain, pale skin, infertility and impotence.

9. "Yin Deficiency" is a red tongue with cracks and little or no coating. Symptoms include night sweats, hot flashes, irritability and insomnia.

10. "Blood Deficiency" is a pale tongue with little or no coating. Symptoms include being dizzy, insomnia, poor memory and fatigue.

The tongue also is a reflection of what is going on in the body, according to TCM. The tongue is divided into sections and each section relates to specific body parts. The tip of your tongue is your heart, and right behind that corresponds to your lungs.

The middle of your tongue on both the left and right side represents your liver and gallbladder and the middle of your tongue in the center represents your stomach and your spleen.

The back of your tongue in the center represents your intestines and bladder and on the sides in the back of your tongue your kidneys are represented.

A simple synopsis would be that a pink-red color tongue indicates good circulation while a purple-colored tongue shows restricted circulation. A pale tongue shows a lack of blood and a tongue which has too much red shows a fever. If a certain spot on the tongue is red it shows unbalance to that corresponding organ in the body.

Your tongue coating can be brushed away but you will notice it does reappear. A healthy body exhibits a thin white coating on the tongue.

Ridges or scallops on the outer edges of the tongue indicate fluid retention. With fluid retention your tongue swells and has no place to rest except against your teeth, causing the imprint from the teeth, or the scalloping, to occur.

In tongue diagnosis the practitioner will check your tongue for movement. A "quivering tongue" may indicate neurological problems.

AYURVEDA

The definition of Ayurveda in Sanskrit translates as "The Science of Life." Ayurveda has its roots in India over 5000 years ago, and some consider Ayurveda to be the oldest of all the healing methods. Herbs and minerals are used and are individually tailored for your own needs. Over 1250 plants are beneficial in Ayurveda medicinal use. It has been documented that these plants are safe and effective in reducing oral bacteria. Ayurveda follows the principle that everyone is made of space, air, fire, water, and earth. When these five elements come together, they mold to three types of energies or doshas. These doshas are called vata, pitta, and kapha. Ayurveda also recognizes that your pattern of energy or constitution stays with you your whole life. When we are out of balance due to trauma and/or emotional states, our constitution is out of balance and steps need to be taken in order to restore the natural state, which is in balance. Vata is known as the energy of movement and is said to be the most powerful of the three doshas. Pitta is known as the energy of digestion and kapha is known as the energy of lubrication. Each person has all of these in their make-up but one is always the strongest. When you are not in a state of balance it is due to the fluctuation of your natural rhythm of these three constitutions. Vata is responsible for muscle and tissue movement and when it is out of sync, fear and anxiety become present. Pitta is in charge of absorption, digestion and body temperature. When Pitta is not in balance, anger presents itself.

Kapha forms bone muscle and tendons in the body and lubricates all of the body. When out of sync the need for attachment becomes prevalent. One main part of an Ayurveda diagnosis is the use of tongue mapping. Also, voice tones and pulse are checked to help diagnose. When checking the color of the tongue it is believed that a white tongue means an imbalance in kapha. A tongue that is either yellow-green or red means an imbalance in pitta, and a brown or black tongue is indicative of vata that is not in balance. A vata tongue is smaller and rough while a pitta tongue is red and medium, and a kappa tongue is fuller light pink and wet. A tongue which is too red and smooth is said to indicate too much stomach acid.

When taste buds react to stress, they hide and thus give your tongue a smooth appearance. Scalloped tongue (teeth marks on the edges) is said to be a result of nutritional imbalance. When a tongue has a thick coating throughout it is said to be the result of improperly digested food. These foods are then congesting the intestinal tract. If the coating is just found on the back of the tongue, it is due to toxins on the large and small intestine as well as the colon. However, if this coating is on the front portion of the tongue, the stomach and small intestine are built up with toxins. A pale tongue can suggest the person is anemic or food isn't being properly digested due to improper amounts of stomach acids and enzymes for proper digestion. Dry tongue is due to lack of proper hydration in the stomach to digest foods.

On the other hand, a wet tongue is an irritated stomach lining due to mucus buildup (kapha), or it can also be caused by an excess of stress. A swollen tongue is caused by congestion in the lymphatic system. Ayurveda teaches that tongue scraping from back to front should be done daily, in the morning and before consuming any foods. It is believed in the practice of Ayurveda that there are 65 types of oral diseases you may get. It is further believed that eight varieties can appear on the lips, fifteen can appear on the alveolar edges, eight have to do with teeth, five can show on the tongue, nine on the palate, seventeen in the oropharynx and three miscellaneously.

Ayurveda does not rely on medicine due to toxicity, but focuses on balancing energy systems in the body. Some basic homecare options in Ayruveda practice include using tea tree oil to help clean gums. Cold sores can heal more quickly by placing aloe vera on them. Coconut oil can be used to help with red gums by massaging into the gum area. Swollen gums are said to be helped by applying turmeric directly on them. When looking for ongoing dental health, Arnia capsules can be taken daily. Collagen stabilization can come from Bilberry Fruit and Hawthorne Berry. To reduce cavities, Liquorice Root is shown to be effective. Ayurveda has been around for thousands of years and is a widely used practice in India for longevity.

AROMATHERAPY

Rene Gattefosse is credited in 1937 with coining the word aromatherapy. He did experimentation with oils and grouped them into the specific modalities of their strengths. These included antitoxic, tonifying, antiseptic, calming and stimulating. Aromatherapy works by affecting your physical and emotional receptors. Once the scents become inhaled, the nasal cavity gets stimulated and sends a signal to the limbic system in the brain. There is then an immediate reaction given off by the circulatory and nervous systems. Everybody reacts differently to the smell of an aromatherapy oil because it is based on memory from a past experience with this same smell. It has been shown that the most unpleasant smell in the dental office is eugenol, which is the oil used in dental fillings. The sense of smell can trigger unpleasant memories and cause anxiety and other feelings. Some other unpleasant dental smells are latex in the gloves, sterilization products, and the smell of a tooth being drilled. One easy way to change the smell in the office, and the negative feelings they may produce, is aromatherapy.

Aromatherapy has been scientifically proven to reduce dental anxiety when using scents such as lavender and/or orange. These two scents have also been proven to boost mood and bring on a sense of calmness. Aromatherapy oils come from different parts of trees and flowers, and are used in small amounts at a time. There are no side effects and it is 100 percent human safe. Some areas where aromatherapy has shown promise in dentistry include toothaches, teething and ulcers, to name a few.

CHAPTER 3
WHAT'S EATING YOU?

TYPES OF TEETH

Teeth start to form in the most basic stage at approximately 6 weeks in utero. Teeth will start to erupt anywhere between 6 and 12 months. Humans have two sets of teeth and this is known as "diphyodont." Baby teeth are also known as milk teeth or primary teeth. "Milk teeth" got its name when it was thought teeth grew due to mother's milk over the gums. "Deciduous teeth," also meaning baby teeth, got its name as teeth were compared to "deciduous trees" which lost their leaves. And since this first set of teeth fall out and get replaced, thus a comparison was made.

"Natal teeth" are any teeth present when a child is born. Many years ago, any child born with a tooth present in their mouth was put to death. It was thought to be a sign they were demons. The exact reason a child would be born with teeth is not clearly known. Certain American Indian tribes do show a higher occurrence of natal teeth. It has also been shown that female infants have a higher incidence of these anomalies.

Lower central incisors (the two teeth in the front middle) make up 85% of natal teeth. The upper central incisors account for 11%, followed by 3% being the lower canines. Sometimes a natal tooth can be sharp and cause an ulcer underneath or on top of the tongue. When underneath the tongue it is a phenomenon known as Riga-Fede syndrome. Natal teeth should be evaluated for mobility (looseness) and possible extraction as to avoid a choking hazard. Sometimes these teeth are supernumerary (extra teeth above the normal number in each arch).

"Neonatal teeth" are any teeth which come in during the first month of a baby's life. The most common neonatal teeth are also the lower central incisors. Rarely will natal and neonatal teeth be present in the same child.

Natal teeth occur three times more than neonatal teeth do. Approximately 15% of children with either of these rarities have a predisposition genetically.

When a full set of primary teeth is erupted there are twenty. There are ten on top and ten of the same corresponding teeth on bottom. The top/upper arch is known as the maxilla or maxillary and the bottom/lower arch is known as the mandible or mandibular arch. By a child's third birthday all twenty primary teeth have erupted in the mouth. A primary dentition consists of central incisors (2 upper 2 lower), lateral incisors (2 upper 2 lower), canines (2 upper 2 lower), and molars (4 upper 4 lower).

Another name which is given to this first set of teeth is "training teeth" as children are training to have good hygiene habits for their second or permanent set of teeth. Since these teeth are normally exfoliated by the age of 12, the name "temporary teeth" can be heard in reference to them. As stated above this first set of teeth to erupt consists of a set of twenty when all are present. By age 3 most toddlers have their full set of primary teeth as above stated.

"Congenitally missing teeth" are any teeth that do not erupt and are not present underneath the gums. Another name for this is "hypotontia." Only one percent of children have been found to have congenitally missing baby teeth. And twenty percent of adults have been found to have congenitally missing permanent teeth. If you are missing more than six of your permanent teeth it is known as "oligodontia." "Anodontia" is when you are missing all of your permanent teeth. On the opposite end of the spectrum is "supernumerary teeth." This is when there are extra teeth (or one extra tooth) present.

Another name given to this extra tooth/ extra teeth phenomenon is "hyerdontia." Permanent teeth are more widely seen with this than primary teeth. Sometimes this is called a third set of teeth. Treatment is determined on an individual basis, based on the occlusion and how much space is available for the tooth in order to not affect bite and spacing. It is more common to have one supernumerary tooth than it is to have many supernumerary teeth. Most of these cases are seen on the upper anterior region of the mouth.

Germination and fused teeth are difficult to tell apart. Germination is also known as double tooth. One root (the part underneath the gumline) is present and the tooth has tried to divide causing two crowns (the part you see outside of the gums). Germination is more prevalent in a primary dentition and is almost always not bilateral. Fusion is also more prevalent in primary teeth, and incisors are most often affected. Fused teeth are two separate tooth germs merging together. This can occur at different stages of tooth development.

"Peg laterals" are also known as Dracula teeth or microdontia. These are anomalies where the tooth is smaller than usual and looks like the shape of a peg. They are easy to fix and are thought to be of congenital nature. In contrast, "macrodontia" includes teeth that are larger than normal size. Megadontia is another name given to teeth that are larger than normal size.

Primary teeth are referred to by their proper names but are also given a universal letter for each tooth. The lettering begins on the upper right molar (the tooth furthest back in the mouth). This upper right molar is letter "A." As you follow the alphabet and the upper arch you will end with the letter "J." This will correlate to the upper left back tooth also known as the second molar. As a side note, if a tooth is not present in the mouth, that tooth still is represented by the correct and proper letter for the tooth. Once on the lower arch you begin with the lower left molar and this is "K." As you complete the lower arch "T" will be the last tooth and will be the lower right second molar.

Humans have two sets of teeth. Once a permanent tooth bud has formed underneath the gums, the root of the corresponding baby tooth begins to resorb. This is what makes teeth loose. It is almost always that the lower central incisors are the first to be loose and replaced. This happens at approximately age 5-6. In a complete set of permanent teeth each arch contains 16 teeth. These teeth are two central incisors, two lateral incisors, two canines, four premolars and six molars. Just as primary teeth have a letter to identify them, permanent teeth have numbers associated with each tooth.

WISDOM TEETH

Starting at the upper right back tooth (third molar or as it is also known, wisdom tooth) is number 1. Continuing around the upper arch until you reach the left third molar/ wisdom tooth is number 16. You then move onto the lower left wisdom tooth which is both 17 and the lower left third molar, and numbers end with the lower right wisdom tooth, number 32, also called lower right third molar. This represents a full set of teeth. There are about 1/3 of the population that never develop wisdom teeth, also known as third molars. Of the people that do get them, sometimes it is advisable to remove them. Some reasons are infection, inhibiting homecare, large areas of decay and cysts. However, studies are being conducted now citing that removing impacted wisdom teeth may not be worth it.

A study was done at the University of York in the UK in 1998. This study concluded there was no evidence backing up removal of otherwise healthy wisdom teeth, whether impacted or erupted. Also, in 1998 the Royal College of Physicians of Edinburgh determined it is not advisable to remove these teeth. Australia and the USA practice the theory that it is better to take wisdom teeth out now than to face a maybe problem later. Some complications of wisdom teeth surgical removal include but are not limited to nerve damage, anesthetic reactions and loss of taste sensation. In the *American Journal of Public Health* Dr. Jay Friedman (an oral surgeon) said it is a "public health hazard" to preventatively remove wisdom teeth. In 2008 the American Public Health Association made a decision to be against preventative wisdom teeth removal.

TONSILS

The same type of findings were found with tonsillectomies. Tonsils are in the back of your throat bilaterally (on both sides). Their job is to keep your immune system strong by filtering germs and keeping infections away. For 30 years children born between 1979 and 1999 were followed in Denmark. Results were published in JAMA (Journal of the American Medical Association) and showed that removal of tonsils increased asthma and upper respiratory infections.

As of the 1980s tonsillectomies are not performed routinely anymore. It was known in Britain as a "dangerous fad." Another study done by University of Birmingham found only 14 percent of children undergoing a tonsillectomy met the prerequisite. Between April 2016 and March 2017, 37000 tonsillectomies were reported. In the UK tonsillectomy guidelines are the removal of tonsils when least seven episodes of sore throats occurred in the previous twelve months period which made the child not well.

It was then found that most of the surgeries were performed on children only having an average of three sore throats per year, not the required seven. A common occurrence in tonsils is tonsil stones otherwise known as "tonsilloliths." It is a white soft or hard bacteria and debris that lands in the crevices of tonsils. Most of the time they go away on their own with no treatment, no side effects and no downtime. If they become large or painful then a doctor visit may be required for removal. A once routine surgery in 1930s for prevention is now realized not to be preventative.

The mouth is forming section by section in utero. Four to seven weeks into pregnancy the lips are being formed. Although cleft lip can show in the middle of the lip, it is mainly on either the right or left side. It may be a small slit but the cleft can reach into the nose. This along with cleft palate is a defect which is the fourth most common type. Cleft lip (unlike cleft palate) may be able to be seen on an ultrasound in utero. The earliest time it can be seen is at week 13 of pregnancy with ultrasounds giving a more definitive reading as pregnancy gets longer. Approximately 81% of cleft lips are diagnosed via ultrasound before birth. Surgery can repair cleft lip with the ideal time being 10-12 weeks of age. There will be a small scar located underneath the nose on the lip area. Neither cleft lip nor cleft palate are life-threatening issues.

LIP LIFTS

There is a proper name for the space between your nose and your mouth. The groove in between your nose and upper lip is known as the "philtrum." As we age this space grows longer in length. The ideal amount between your nose and the border of your upper lip is 1.1-1.2 cm or 11-13 mm. This is the mark that someone is considered attractive. The philtrum has no purpose and does vary in length person to person. Lips that are noticed have three common factors and this spacing is one of them. Other factors include fullness and a cupid's bow that is defined. Cupid's bow is the middle part of your upper lip where it dips down. Surgical and non-surgical lip lifts are offered for a long philtrum.

As people age the ligaments giving the face support weaken and get looser, causing the structures to be thinner, and the philtrum to become longer. It is estimated that for every ten years after your twenties, the philtrum drops 1-3 mm. A lip lift also lets more of the front teeth show, which is a sign of youthfulness. Stitches are in place for about a week after this procedure.

Two popular types of lip lift surgeries are known as "The Direct Vermillion or Gulwing Lip Lift" and "The Subnasal Bullhorn Lip Lift." And there are different variations that each plastic surgeon has created to be their signature lip lift. In a surgical lip lift the upper lip is made to look more youthful and also fuller. There is a scar underneath your nose which is where the incision is made. Anesthesia is required for this procedure. Lip lifts are considered cosmetic, and insurance companies will not cover the fee, which could be one deterrent. Surgical lip lifts are permanent and they cost a lot, which could also deter one from having the procedure. There is a scar, though hidden underneath the nose.

Some people do not opt for lip lifts. There are options available that do not involve surgery and are also not permanent. Getting lip filler is temporary and a very common and accepted practice. One type of temporary filler option is "hyaluronic acid." HA is produced in your body and is a natural substance. HA is used in skincare because it plumps the skin and keeps it plump. HA can hold up to 1000 times its weight in water. This material is also known to look natural. At first expect your lips to be swollen but that swelling disappears over a couple of days. HA filler lasts approximately 6 - 12 months.

On the rare occasion that you do not like your filler, a substance can be injected that will erase and dissolve it. Sometimes, small bumps can be felt when lips are filled, but they can be massaged to blend in better. Some benefits to HA injections include short treatment time, no downtime and mild to no side effects. The downside to lip fillers is that they can look "like a duck," bruising can occur, and filler can be lumpy and need to repeated frequently to keep lips looking full and plump.

Another option for making lips fuller is fat injections. Fat injections are also known as grafting. Liposuction is done on another part of the body then the fat is transferred to the lips. Benefits of this include a natural look as it is your own fat, long-lasting results and no incisions to the face. Some downsides to fat transfer are need for anesthesia, uneven liposuction risks, and healing time is approximately 2 weeks.

Another choice is a lip implant. Lip implants are mainly used when wanting a noticeable size increase. Lip implants are a permanent solution. Small incisions, which are hidden in lip corners, are used to put the implant into place. This is usually done under local anesthesia. Benefits to a lip implant include long-lasting results, only a couple days of downtime, and short procedure time. Some risk factors are incision scars, uneven lips, and cost.

Lip augmentation is ever increasing and 2016 saw a 53% increase from 2000 (28,500 lip enhancements were performed in 2016).

BOTOX

Botox is used for and not limited to migraines, TMJ pain, crow's feet, forehead lines and for a gummy smile. In order to reduce the amount of gum showing when someone smiles, the botox is injected above the smile at a point known as "Yonsei Point." Ideally one centimeter from the bottom edge of your nose toward your ear and 3 cm up from the edge of your upper lip is the point known as "Yonsei Point." Botox works by paralyzing muscles and in a gummy smile this prevents the lips from opening on top and exposing a lot of gum. HA plumps and sometimes these two are used simultaneously. This will give you approximately 4-6 months of a smile which doesn't show as much gum tissue. While 14% of woman show more than 4 mm of gum when smiling (definition of gummy smile), only 7% of men have this characteristic. An ideal smile has less than 2mm of gum showing.

Some pros on using botox to help a gummy smile include almost immediate results, no downtime and no anesthesia. Some cons include the fact that repeated visits are needed as botox is temporary, possible allergic reaction and if too much is injected it inhibits lip movement and looks unnatural. (A permanent solution to gummy smiles are gum lifts also known as gingivectomy or crown lengthening. In this procedure gum tissue adjacent to teeth is cut to expose the tooth and make the tooth longer.)

Botox can be beneficial for issues that are not cosmetic. Botox is also effective for clenching and grinding habits. When used in this type of situation botox can last 3-5 months. Botox is injected into the masseter muscles and also the temporals muscles. Grinding and clenching can be caused by stress, an abnormal bite, misaligned teeth, sleep apnea, etc. Approx. 1/3 of children grind their teeth and sometimes no one is aware of it. Dental professionals can look at occlusal wear patterns and help determine of you are in fact grinding. Of the children that do grind, most of them stop by the time they are teenagers.

NIGHTGUARDS

Nightguards have been shown to help with grinding and or clenching as they take pressure off the teeth. You are biting into the plastic and saving your teeth from contact with each other. This contact leads to the wear and can make the tooth smaller as you grind it away. Nightguards can be purchased from your dental office or you can purchase them over the counter.

There are some factors to consider when opting for a night guard through a dental office vs over the counter. It is much more expensive to get a nightguard made in the office rather than over the counter. Instructions may be confusing at home so you may want to get a professional one made. Getting a nightguard made in a dental office will fit better, as a mold of your teeth is used. However, if you do one on your own you do not wait until the lab has finished making yours, you can make your own instantly. Nightguards can be made of hard plastic, soft plastic or a combination where soft plastic is on the inside and hard plastic is on the outside.

Feel free to wear your nightguard during the day if you find yourself clenching and or grinding not only at night. Some other issues arising with nightguards may include tender gums, funny taste in mouth and more saliva than normal.

The roof of the mouth is known as the palate and forms between six and nine weeks into pregnancy. Sometimes the mouth does not completely close and thus results in a cleft palate. As stated above, cleft palate is not life-threatening. Surgery can be performed at approximately 9-12 months.

A cleft palate does involve both the hard and soft tissues of the palate (roof of the mouth). It is said that African babies have the lowest incidence of a cleft and that Asian babies have the highest occurrence. Eating and/or speaking does become a problem when cleft lip and or cleft palate is present. Cleft lip and cleft palate are a very common birth defect and their origin is unknown.

Surgery is often recommended to repair these defects and it has been shown to be beneficial within the first 18 months of life. The sooner the surgery is done the better for the child, with some surgeries being performed as early as one week of age. It has been found that only 20 percent of cleft lips and palates are inherited. If left untreated, a cleft can interfere with eating, speaking, and breathing. If a child is born with both a cleft lip and a cleft palate, it is known as "orofacial cleft."

Mamelons are not always present in a primary dentition but are always present in permanent central and lateral incisors. Mamelons are a set of three rounded edges on the biting surface of these teeth. They are present from eruption until they get worn away. The edges get worn down by biting and chewing and do not take long to disappear. In an open bite the edges will remain rounded and obvious.

Besides these mamelons/edges on teeth, there are five surfaces. They are known as mesial (front), distal (back), occlusal (top), buccal also known as facial (outside) and lingual (inside). When talking about the gum joining the tooth area, that is referred to as the gingival. Anterior teeth are considered the central incisors, lateral incisors and canines. Posterior teeth consist of premolars and molars. There are several types of occlusions, also known as "bites." Class I is a "normal" or preferred bite where first molars line up in a certain fashion and upper teeth slightly overlap lower teeth. Class II is known as a malocclusion since is not the standard bite. Class II occurs when the upper teeth overlap the lower teeth in a severe manner. As a side note, the difference between overbite as in this case and overjet is as follows. An overbite is the vertical relationship of upper to lower teeth. Upper teeth should cover the lower teeth 1/3 to 1/2 of the way in order to not be considered this. However, most people have some degree of an overbite and unless severe won't cause any issues. Overjet is measured by the horizontal protrusion of upper teeth to lower teeth.

A lot of overjet occlusions are due to habits such as tongue thrust or nail biting. Some other types of "bites" which are seen include an open bite. This is where the anterior teeth are not touching. This type of bite puts extra pressure on posterior teeth. Crossbite is another one which is seen. This is where the lower teeth are outside of the upper teeth when biting down. Crossbite can involve any one tooth or can involve many teeth. It can also be unilateral, but is not always. Spacing and crowding are other types of odontology. It is important to know that when primary dentition has spacing this is a good sign. When permanent teeth erupt, they are larger than primary teeth and the primary spacing gives them room to grow in at a good angle. Class III occlusion is also known as underbite. This is when the lower anterior teeth are in front of the upper anterior tech when closing. Another term for Class III occlusion is "prognathism."

WHAT YOU SHOULD KNOW ABOUT LIPSTICK

Did you know that certain lipstick shades can enhance your teeth and make them appear whiter? For example, if your teeth are grey (which could be from taking tetracycline while teeth were forming), wear pink or a berry shade of lipstick. If your teeth are yellow, wear a warm peach or nude shade of lipstick. These will make your teeth appear whiter. Lipstick has been around for approximately 5000 years. Social status was shown by both Egyptian men and women wearing lipstick . Red lipstick is known as a symbol of empowerment and dates back to Mesopotamia, approximately 3500 B.C.E. It was there and then that red rocks were turned into powder by crushing them. Red is known to symbolize love. The first tube of lipstick was made of metal and invented in 1915. A lever on the side moved the lipstick up and down. Maurice Levy gets the credit for this invention. There are some tips and tricks to make lipstick coloring work best for you and your teeth. As a general rule wear cool toned lipstick if you'd like your teeth to appear whiter. Orange, brown and neon shades of lipstick will tend to show the yellow shading in teeth. Nude or peach tones will also give your teeth a yellow hue. A blue undertone pink lipstick is best for making teeth appear whiter. A yellow undertone in a pink lipstick will make the teeth appear to be more yellow. If you prefer to wear red lipstick, opt for a blue tone to bring out the white in your teeth. If you pick an orange tone you will notice your teeth looking more yellow, but if you pick the pink toned red lipstick it won't change your teeth to the naked eye. The darker the lip color shade, the more yellow your teeth will seem to be. Lipsticks are made with wax and alcohol, amongst other ingredients. However, some lipsticks do contain lead. Lipsticks are not the only cosmetics on the market with lead in them. Lead exposure from lipstick comes mainly from licking one's lips. The FDA has determined that 10ppm (parts per million) is a safe amount to have in lipstick, although some people say no amount is safe due to the buildup over time. Lead is a neurotoxin linked to fertility problems and learning issues to name a few. An FDA investigation in 2010 found lead over 7ppm in 400 lipsticks. Lead won't be listed on the ingredients nor will some other toxins found in lipstick investigations. The University of California did a study finding aluminum, cadmium and manganese in lipsticks investigated. These are all heavy metals. The Campaign for Safe Cosmetics has determined through their study that there are several brands of lipstick that contain no lead. They are currently sold and do have a wide range of price points.

CHAPTER 4
DOES MILK DO A BODY GOOD?

Remember the TV commercial that said milk does a body good and milk builds strong teeth and bones? Although it was thought that calcium was the element for strong bones, magnesium has now been proven to allow a strong skeleton. The Pediatric Academic Society is suggesting magnesium as well as calcium be considered. Too much calcium has been shown to increase heart attacks and is a risk for kidney stones. Calcium supplements do not get to the bone structure, and since calcium is hard to excrete, it finds its way to other areas of the body. The plaque from the calcium accumulates in arteries and inhibits blood flow. This is especially true for females and for those using calcium supplements. The Mayo Clinic does support that calcium can be found in other items besides milk and it is acceptable to do so. Some common slogans present day are "Not your mother ,not your milk" and "You need calcium not milk."

WHAT IS IN OUR MILK?

There are several types of calcium including calcium carbonate, calcium citrate, calcium lactate, calcium gluconate and calcium citrate malate. Only 500 mg of calcium can be absorbed by the body at one time so anything taken over that amount is not used in the body. You need to have enough vitamin D in order to absorb the calcium into your system.

Calcium from oyster shell, bone meal, dolomite and/or coral may have toxic metals and/or lead in them and it is not recommended to take these. Negative interactions can occur when taking calcium supplements at the same time as iron supplements, zinc supplements, tetracycline (antibiotic), or levothyroxine (hypothyroid drug). It is recommended to wait several hours in between.

Calcium carbonate, also known as an antacid, needs stomach acid to work so one should eat with this type of calcium. "Tums" is an example of calcium carbonate. No more than 7500 mg a day should be consumed. Calcium carbonate is contraindicated in people with kidney stones or low phosphate blood levels. It is also not advisable if you take Lanoxin, Cardoxin or Digitek. The FDA puts calcium carbonate in the 'C' category. What this means is that the effects on an unborn baby are unclear. It is not recommended to breastfeed and take calcium carbonate. It passes through breast milk and is considered safe though not recommended. Side effects do include, but are not limited to, dizziness, nausea, constipation and stomach distention. Serious side effects of calcium carbonate include kidney stones, low blood phosphate levels and high blood calcium levels. If these occur a doctor should be notified immediately. It is recommended to not take calcium carbonate if you take the drug Rocephin. Antifungal medications such as Nizoral can interact with calcium carbonate, as well as certain antibiotics. If you are taking any medications discuss with your doctor before taking. While taking calcium carbonate, the chance of stomach irritation can be increased if alcohol is consumed. This type of calcium is the most widespread and can't be fully absorbed without something like citric acid. Calcium carbonate is in pasteurized milk as well.

Calcium lactate should be taken with food. Effervescent tablets need to be fully dissolved in water and not taken whole or chewed. Liquid calcium lactate should be measured exactly. The same precautions and side effects of calcium lactate apply to the others listed.

Calcium gluconate is administered via IV at 100mg/ml. It is also available in a tablet or capsule form. This type of calcium is indicated in for hypocalcemia tetany, hypocalcemia from hypoparathyroidism and hypocalcemia during pregnancy. Ceftriaxone is on the list of severe drug interactions. Tetracycline, doxycycline, minocycline, and oxytetracycline are some of the drugs on the serious interaction list. It has been shown that calcium gluconate has moderate interactions with over 50 drugs and has mild interactions with over 50 drugs as well. There are some warnings associated with this type of calcium that include but are not limited to the following… Use with caution in pregnancy. Animal testing does show risks. Cardiac arrest may occur.

Calcium citrate can cause lack of urination and weight gain. Nausea, vomiting and muscle weakness are some symptoms of too much calcium in your system. Calcium citrate can be taken with or without food. Pills should not be broken or crushed as they may be extended release. Chewable tablets are to be chewed thoroughly. It is possible to get an upset stomach or constipation. A doctor should be notified if you experience nausea or vomiting, loss of appetite, mood changes, urination changes, increase in thirst or rapid heartbeat, to name a few. Calcium citrate does come mixed with vitamin D as well as magnesium.

Plants do contain calcium and have been said to be the best source of it. You can achieve your daily calcium level without the consumption of dairy. Here are some examples of foods rich in calcium: chia seeds, sesame seeds, spinach, turnip greens, kale, broccoli, bok choy, and pumpkin seeds, just to name a few.

Lactose is a sugar which is in dairy. Lactose intolerance or the inability to digest this sugar is a common ailment. In the US over 3 million people a year are found to have this. Lactose intolerance has no cure but changing diet can help alleviate symptoms. Common symptoms of lactose intolerance include pain in the abdomen, diarrhea and or constipation.

Another common allergy is to casein. Casein is a protein found in milk. A blood test can determine if you have a casein allergy and should avoid dairy.

Magnesium has recently become a big topic as far as bone health is concerned. It is just as important for pediatrics as it is for the elderly. Since the 1950s the magnesium in soil has gone down approximately 40% and produce has declined in magnesium almost 80%. This is due to the demand for fast crops. Almonds, cashews, cacao, chia seeds and sesame seeds are just some of the foods containing a high level of magnesium. Magnesium when supplementing is absorbed more at nighttime and can be taken with or without food. The recommended daily allowance is 350-400 mg/day. It is difficult to measure readings of magnesium on blood tests due to your body storing it in the blood then sending to the bones when they need to be replenished.

Vitamin D3 is important as it aids in calcium absorption. Most people are deficient in Vitamin D3, and levels can be measured on a blood test. Vitamin K2 as well as phosphorous are also important in calcium absorption.

The issue of dairy necessity and safety has been raised lately. It has been said that cow's milk is not fit for human consumption. Human milk has 1/3 the protein of cow's milk and has been said to offset metabolism. Dairy is an inflammatory food and produces mucus. Allergies are increased and the possibility of respiratory issues rises. Kidney stones can be caused by dairy, due to the excess calcium which needs to exit the body.

America has a very high rate of osteoporosis and also the highest rate of daily consumption. Osteoporosis doesn't allow for the new bone to be created in direct response to the old bone being removed. Bodies are doing this constantly and so the bones become brittle. There is treatment for osteoporosis but there is no cure. Over 3 million people are diagnosed with osteoporosis every year. Early stages of osteoporosis have no symptoms.

THE DOWNSIDES OF DRINKING COW'S MILK

Some things that are present in cow's milk which raise concern are pus, antibiotics, cholesterol, bovine growth hormone and feces, just to name a few. The acidic animal protein that is also in cow's milk is said to pull calcium from the bones. There have been published reports linking cow's milk to colic, salmonella, allergic reactions, sinusitis and heart disease. For people opting not to drink cow's milk, whether they are vegans or lactose intolerant or otherwise, there are approximately twenty-five foods which have more calcium than a glass of milk pound for pound. Dairy is not the only source of calcium.

The Centre for Science in the Public Interest and the Wall Street Journal sampled milk in ten cities. Their findings were that 38% of the samples were contaminated with antibiotics and/or sulfa drugs. A study similar to this was done in Washington DC, and found 20% of milk sampled to be contaminated.

The Cohort of Sweden has found that drinking three or more glasses of milk per day increased cardiovascular mortality vs drinking less than one glass per day of milk.

Lactose intolerant individuals consuming milk get diarrhea, which can lead to loss of protein.

Over 20,000 male doctors participated in the Harvard's Physicians Health Study. It was found that the ones that ingested two or more dairy servings per day increased their risk of prostate cancer by 34% over those having no dairy or very minimal dairy daily.

Galctose is in lactose (milk sugar) and has possibly been linked in studies to ovarian cancer. One glass of milk contains approximately 10 grams of lactose.

Ovarian cancer increases 13% per each 10 grams consumed. This was reported by The Physicians Committee for Responsible Medicine.

Many studies have been documented concluding that cow's milk consumed by infants and toddlers interferes with iron stores. When cow's milk is iron fortified it can help with the iron status and protect from negativity. Unfortified cow's milk is not recommended for infants and should only be used sparingly for toddlers.

Yale University School of Medicine studied the correlation between cow's milk and dairy as they relate to hip fractures in women over 50 years of age. America has the highest milk consumption, only behind Australia, New Zealand and Europe. As suspected, the higher the milk consumption the higher incidence of hip fracture. The University of California San Francisco studied women over 64 for seven years. Over 1000 women participated and it was found that those who consumed higher animal protein than plant protein increased their incidence of bone fractures.

Pus is in your milk. One million cells per spoonful of concentrated pus. The U.S. dairy industry will tell you that having pus in dairy is not bad because the animals have a defense system which pus is part of. They also say that since milk is pasteurized it is okay and not a safety concern. When cow udders are infected inflamed, they are still milked.

Flavoring milk is not beneficial from the sugar standpoint for one. Calcium absorption is lessened with sugar.

IMPORTANT DATES IN MILK HISTORY

It is speculated that the first cattle used for human consumption by milking was by Neolithic farmers in Britain and Northern Europe. Humans were first able to digest milk around 4500 B.C.E. This was due to "lactase persistence" which is a genetic mutation. In approximately 300 B.C.E. milking cows was a part of Sumerian civilization. Not only did they drink milk but they also made dairy products such as cheese and butter. New England saw its first cows in 1624 at Plymouth Rock.

"Cowpox" is a caused by a virus that is transferable from animal to human, and otherwise known as a "zoonotic' virus. Dairymaids milking infected cows would break out in pustules on their hands. It was in the late 1700s that this was seen. Cowpox does resemble smallpox but is milder. It was also discovered that the infected dairymaids were immune to smallpox. Smallpox disappeared by the 1980s.Cowpox is also seen in rodents, and is now believed they were responsible for the transfer to humans.

Pasteurization was developed by Louis Pasteur, a French chemist and biologist in the 1800s. He discovered that sickness was caused by milk's harmful microbes. The pasteurization process involves rapidly heating then cooling liquid in order to kill most of the germs.

Dr. Henry Thatcher patented one of the first glass milk bottles in 1884. Glass was the standard for milk, as was the milkman delivery, until the 1950s when waxed paper cartons made their debut.

Milk was known to spread tuberculosis and typhoid when the production was not hygienic. And the mid to late 1800s had a big problem with milk-born illness. Dr. Henry Coit, M.D. had a son die from contaminated milk. In

1893 he formed a "Medical Milk Commission" to certify cleanliness in milk production.

The United States first saw commercial pasteurization machines for milk in 1895.

Auguste Gaulin patented his milk homogenizer in 1899. Homogenization occurs once the large globules of fat are broken down to smaller ones. Unhomogenized milk has cream that rises to the top.

Typhoid was rampant in New York City and contaminated milk was to blame.

The encouragement of milk pasteurization began in 1917. Cows proven to not have tuberculosis were the exception to the rule.

In 1937 BST proves to increase milk production in cattle.

June 4, 1940 marks the anniversary of federal assistance milk programs. Chicago was where this began, and was capped at 15 elementary schools. These schools were all in low-income neighborhoods. Donations helped the children who could not pay, and those who could afford to pay were charged one cent for a half pint of milk.

The "National School Lunch Act" was signed into law 1946 by President Harry Truman. Lunches for the entire nation would be provided and of good nutritional value. Although there were three types of lunches, Type A, Type B and Type C, all were to provide 1/2 to 2 pints of whole milk.

The introduction of paper cartons in the 1950s allowed for more cost-effectiveness over glass bottles. Paper was cheaper than glass and more product could take up less room.

"The Child Nutrition Act of 1966" allowed the "Special Milk Program." President Lyndon B. Johnson signed this law and it provided free or reduced-fee milk at school to those places not in the other programs.

Once the FDA required that foods have nutritional information on each product, milk got nutritional labeling. This happened in 1974.

The "Dairy Production Stabilization Act of 1983" was a national self-help program. It allowed for promotion and nutritional education on milk packaging in order to make human milk as well as dairy consumption higher.

Biotechnology in the 1980s allows for large quantities of bST production. bST is Bovine somatotropin - a growth hormone.

In 1990 the "Fluid Milk Promotion Act" has the purpose of the promotion of milk sales and milk advertising. The Fluid Milk Promotion Act stood by the belief milk is a worthwhile basic food and beneficial source of calcium for human consumption. The Act mandated that the availability of milk products is important to ensure that the US population is receiving proper nutrition.

The U.S.D.A. (United States Department of Agriculture) exhibited the first food pyramid in 1992. Its hope was to educate people to make good or better nutritional choices. This food pyramid recommends 2-3 servings of dairy per day.

In 1993, the "California Milk Processor Board" was launched to increase the intake of milk. Their slogan became "Got Milk?""Got Milk" is known as one of the most persuasive advertising campaigns to date, with the dairy industry spending almost $15 million dollars annually in support.

"Got Milk" became a federal trademark and went national in 1995.

November 5, 1993 rBST, rBGH, BGH - genetically modified artificial cattle hormone was approved by the FDA for commercial usage in United States.

In 1993 "Posilac" (a bST product) was FDA approved for use in dairy cows. Although some side effects were noted in these cows, the FDA calls the side effects manageable..

In 1994 protests began around the country in response to the use of artificial bovine growth hormone in milk. The organizer of the Pure Food Campaign, Jeremy Rifkin, thought the was a health hazard. Also, in 1994, the FDA had a new guideline for rBST. Dairy products from cows that were not given the artificial bovine growth hormone rBST required a disclaimer on the label. It was to state, "No significant difference has been shown between milk derived from rbST-treated and non-rbST-treated cows."

The Dairy Management, Inc. formed in 1995,and made up of board members from the National Dairy Board and the United Dairy Industry. It is their responsibility to increase the need for dairy products produced in the USA. The U.S. Dairy Export Council is formed by the Dairy Management Inc and it is in place to "leverage investments of dairy processors, exporters, dairy producers, and industry suppliers to enhance the U.S. dairy industry ability to serve international markets."

Mattel and "Got Milk?"partnered then released a limited edition "Got Milk?" barbie in 1995. Its goal was for young people to be encouraged to drink milk.

In 1997 a very important study was published in the *American Journal of Public Health*. The study was done by doctors at Harvard School of Public Health, and was called "Milk, Dietary Calcium, and Bone Fractures in Women: A 12- Year Prospective Study." This study investigated the role of higher calcium and milk products in adults as it related to the risk of bone fractures and osteoporosis. The study found "high intakes of milk (two or more glasses a day over a 12-year period did not reduce the incidence of osteoporosis and related bone fractures."

In 1998 the Weston A. Price Foundation started the "Real Milk Campaign." It was to show positive benefits for health by consuming raw cow's milk and to get the sale of raw cow's milk approved not only in the USA but worldwide. Seventeen US states in 2007 determined selling raw cow's milk for human usage was illegal.

December 2001 marked the time Dean Foods was acquired by Suiza Foods. With $10 billion dollars in revenue and over 25,000 workers, the new Dean Foods is at that time the largest processor of dairy in the nation.

In December 2002 the California Milk Advisory Board was sued by PETA (People for the Ethical Treatment of Animals). They sued in regard to the "Happy Cows" advertising, calling it false. The picture of the cows being happy instead of showing the real living conditions was the basis of the lawsuit. In 2002 the California Superior Court rejects the lawsuit and in 2005 they deny the appeal by PETA.

January 5, 2004 is the date Horizon Organic was acquired by Dean Foods. Horizon Organic was the number one organic processor of dairy.

In 2004 was when the "3-A-Day. Burn More Fat, Lose Weight" campaign was released. The message was that weight loss could be faster by consuming 3 dairy servings each day. The campaign was started by the National Dairy Promotion and Research Board along with Dairy Management, Inc. This ad could be seen on the internet, television and in print.

2005 saw a 23 percent increase in organic milk intake over 2004, and an 8 percent decrease overall in the intake of milk. Also, in 2005 the Dietary Guidelines for Americans were updated to state, "Consume 3 cups per day of fat-free or low-fat milk or equivalent milk products." This was done by the United States Department of Agriculture and the Department of Health and Human Services. In October of this year a class action lawsuit was filed by the Physicians Committee for Responsible Medicine (PCRM) representing every resident of Washington, D.C. It was to make sure warnings were present on milk in regard to lactose intolerance. The lawsuit was "to help raise public awareness about lactose intolerance… on behalf of all residents in Washington D.C. who may purchase milk without realizing the serious digestive distress it can cause." Filed in the Superior Court of the District of Columbia on October 6, the suit called for all milk cartons sold in D.C. to carry labels warning of milk's possible side effects.

Milk intake continued to decline in Japan and surplus milk became an issue. In one month alone Hokkaido needed to get rid of 900 tons of extra milk. Chitoshi Nakahara is a liquor store owner in Hokkaido who takes advantage, experiments and ferments surplus milk. "Bilk" becomes the beer he creates and in 2007 "Bilk" was being sold in liquor stores locally.

In 2007 the claims supporting weight loss with milk were withdrawn. Any and all marketing of this claim and advertising was ceased.

In 2007 the largest producer of organic milk was Aurora Organic Dairy. On April 16, 2007 they received a letter from the USDA with 14 violations they had committed. Some stores supplied by Aurora Organic Dairy included Target, Costco, Safeway and Walmart.

Monsanto Corporation filed a complaint with the Federal Trade Commission in February 2007. Monsanto said their milk is not inferior even with rBST and artificial growth hormone. The response from the FTC is as follows. Its "staff agrees with the FDA that food companies may inform consumers in advertising, as in labeling, that they do not use rBST."

In 2008 a scandal involving tainted milk in China was exposed. At least six children died, and close to 300,000 others got sick when poisoned milk was sold. The company boss got a sentence of life in prison and two men got the death penalty for their roles. Sanlu baby formula was laced with melamine, which is a fertilization chemical. The milk was distributed to dairies after it was watered down and purchased from farmers. Kidney problems in over 50,000 was one result of the melamine. In 2008 recalls were called into action worldwide when melamine appeared in foods such as chocolate and yogurt.

January 8, 2008 marks the day the FDA approved milk from cloned species. Their document informed consumers food and drink from cloned animals and or their offspring were no less safe than traditionally bred animals.

On August 3, 2011 James Cecil Stewart, Sharon Ann Palmer and Eugenie Bloch were arrested for allegedly selling and producing unpasteurized dairy.

"Rawesome Foods" was the market in Venice, California operated by James Cecil Stewart.

"Healthy Family Farms" was run by Sharon Ann Palmer, and Eugenie Bloch was an employee at this location.

The report titled "Non-pasteurized dairy products, Disease Outbreaks, and State Laws - United States 1993-1996" was released by the CDC in March 2012. The conclusion was as follows: "Public health officials at all levels should continue to develop innovative methods to educate consumers and caregivers about the dangers associated with non-pasteurized dairy products. State officials should consider further restricting or prohibiting the sale or distribution of non-pasteurized dairy products to consumers. Consumption of non-pasteurized dairy products cannot be considered safe under any circumstances."

On February 24, 2014 "Milk Life" replaced the "Got Milk?" slogan. Around this time protein was a big news item, and "Milk Life" emphasized that milk also had a nutritional benefit protein. This was in effort to raise declining milk sales by the Milk Processor Education Program.

There was a 7 percent decline in the sale of dairy milk in 2015, which equated to a loss of 17.8 billion dollars. The hypothesis was that another 11 percent drop would be seen over the next five years. However, the sale of non-dairy milk products increased by 9 percent in 2015, which equated to 1.9 billion dollars.

There is a difference of opinion on whether non-dairy milk should actually be called "milk." A judge ruled that soy milk can be called soy milk as consumers realize the difference in soy milk and dairy milk.

On June 1, 2016, Made by Cow, a company in Sydney, Australia, got the okay to sell "Cold Pressure Processing." This was to be instead of heat pasteurization and was approved by the NSW Food Authority. Mr. Joye was the company founder and said water pressure would ensure that no harmful micro-organisms would be present. Micro-organisms presented more risk of a serious illness, and were the reason raw milk selling was illegal in Australia. "Cold Pressed Raw Milk" was not seen as raw due to the high pressure processing it had to go through. The product was studied for over a year to ensure its safety.

In 2017 sales of milk were approximately 14.7 billion dollars and in 2018 they had dropped to 13.6 billion dollars.

The sale of Oat Milk reached 53 million dollars in 2019, which was a 636% increase over 2018.

It was projected that over 18 billion dollars was to be spent on milk alternative products in 2019.

Milk intake has decreased over the last 50 years by about 40 percent. In order to produce milk consistently, dairy cows are bred every year. Calves are taken away from the mothers very quickly and the mothers are calling for them and looking for their babies.

Elmhurst Milked is a farm in New York that now uses plant-based milk rather than dairy cows. Items such as nuts, oats and rice are used to make milk products. Jay Wilde of the UK took over his father's dairy farm upon his father's death in 2011. Jay had become a vegetarian at age 26. He stopped producing dairy because he could not bear to separate the calves from their mothers, which was common practice.

Jan Gerdes of North Germany was a dairy farmer who turned his farm into a sanctuary.

"Michelle" of Israel gave up dairy farming due to the traumatic things she had witnessed. She encourages everyone to not drink dairy or eat animals.

Chris Mills is a former dairy farmer who also became vegan and turned his farm into a sanctuary.

Giacomazzi Dairy farm is now growing almonds instead of doing dairy. This is California's oldest dairy farm and has been in existence for 125 years.

T. Colin Campbell is a biochemist who advocates a plant-based diet. He is the co-author with his son of *The China Study*, which looks at the correlation of animal product intake and chronic diseases. His conclusion is that "people who eat a whole foods, plant based diet - excluding all animal products - can avoid, reduce, and in many cases reverse the development of numerous illnesses, including most of the leading fatal western diseases." When he did this research, he was under the impression that protein from animal sources was essential for a healthy diet. It is his finding and belief that "casein, the main protein in milk and dairy products, is the most significant carcinogen we consume."

A recent survey of teenage vegetarians and vegans showed that these teens chose their diet for both health reasons and animal cruelty prevention. From 2006 to 2016 there was a 350% increase in vegans in the U.K. And almost half of these fall are 15-34 years of age. The years 1993 to 2018 saw an increase in vegan and vegetarian restaurants, from 55 to 971. This was in the USA as well as Canada. "Veganuary" is when people are vegan the month of January. The year 2018 saw 168,500 people participating, representing growth of 183%. The year 2017 had 59,500 people participating.

On November 12, 2019 Dean Foods filed for Chapter 11 bankruptcy. Because Dean Foods was so huge in the dairy market, this makes you think.

CHAPTER 5
LET'S GET TO THE ROOT OF IT

ROOT CANAL THERAPY

Root canal .... a deep-rooted problem and filled with controversy. What is a "root canal?" Why are teeth the only dead thing in a body to be saved? Many doctors and many researchers are following the lead of Dr. Weston Price. He was one of the first to see the link between illness and root canal therapy. It has been shown in studies that much bacteria can still be alive after sodium hypochlorite treats the tooth.

Root Canal is the removal of the nerve and the pulp from a tooth. The root or roots of the tooth is cleaned out and subsequently sealed. The pulp is the inside layer of a tooth which is covered by dentin and that in turn is covered by enamel. Some symptoms which would lead a dentist to determine you need a root canal are an abscess on your gum, a severely broken tooth, decay close to your nerve and an abscess on the root of the tooth (which would be seen on a dental X-ray).

Dr. Stuart Nunnally DDS, MS led a study as reported in *The Truth About Cancer*. Eighty-seven patients with RCT were studied and they all had the same results. Everyone had decreased health within three years of their RCT.

Dr. Josef Issels has been specializing in cancer for over 40 years, and is the author of the book *Cancer: A Second Opinion*. Part of his treatment plan involves removing all RCT teeth. He believes there is a correlation between RCT causing cancer and other diseases.

A general dentist can perform root canal treatments, often abbreviated and referred to as RCT. However, there is a group of dentists known as endodontists who specialize in performing RCT. The definition of endodontics is "inside the tooth." An endodontist first finishes dental school, then continues for two more years of training. During these two years they concentrate on issues relating to the inside structure of the teeth. An endodontist on average will finish 25 RCTs in one week as compared to a general dentist who will complete on average 2 RCTs in one week.

Over 40,000,000 root canals are performed in the USA every year. There are also a few types of surgery that an endodontist performs but the bulk of their practice is performing RCT. The nerve of each tooth is in the canals of every tooth and when an RCT is done, this nerve is removed thus removing pain. The root of your tooth remains in place. Once a root canal is done, the tooth is more fragile than before. The only "job" of the nerves in your teeth is to provide you with the cold and hot sensations that you feel. A tooth can function with or without a nerve. However, once a nerve is removed from a tooth is considered to not be a live tooth anymore and is known as a dead tooth. The steps to a root canal and simple and for the most part uniform.

A dental X-ray will be evaluated to first determine the need for RCT and then to determine how many canals to the tooth has and see the shapes etc. Next you will be given a local anesthetic oil order to avoid pain. Lidocaine is the anesthetic of choice. Topical jelly may or may not be placed on the gum tissue before the injection. Topical jelly will numb the gum in order to reduce the pain on site of injection. Local dental anesthetics do come with and without epinephrine. Epinephrine is a vasoconstrictor and lets the anesthesia last longer. Epinephrine is also known as adrenaline. Some side effects of epinephrine anesthetic include but are not limited to increased heart rate, increased blood pressure and flushed skin.

When doing a root canal, it is especially important that the tooth remain dry so a "rubber dam" is placed around the tooth to isolate it and keep the dryness intact. The dryness reduces bacteria and saliva from entering the tooth to be treated. Rubber dams are also known as a dental dam and is 6 inches of thin square material. The common materials this is made from are latex and nitrile (gloves are also made from these two materials).

Sanford Christie Barnum came up with the idea in 1864. Bacteria, decay and debris are excavated from the root. This is done by drilling a hole and using endodontic files. These files vary in size and the smaller ones are used first. They scrape the sides of the root to make sure it is totally clear of any infection. Periodically water will get flushed in to clear out debris. After clearing out the tooth, it must be sealed. Some dentists choose to fill the tooth right after the RCT, while other dentists wait 7-10 days. Gutta percha (a rubbery material) is commonly used inside a root canal tooth to seal it. A temporary filling seals the access hole to the root and a crown should ultimately be placed on an RCT tooth.

The first root canal instrument was said to be made in 1838 from a watch spring. It is believed that gold foil or asbestos was used to fill pulp chambers until gutta percha was used beginning around 1847. Gutta percha is still used today by both endodontists and general dentists to fill pulp chambers in a root canal procedure.

Having a tooth with RCT makes the tooth more brittle, thus requiring a "crown" also known as a "cap." A crown is made to mimic your tooth shape size and color, assuming you are not changing these features. First your tooth will be prepped (ground down) and an impression will be made for the lab to make the final crown. Sometimes these teeth will need a post and core or possibly only a core. A core is used when the tooth does not have much structure left. This could be caused by extensive decay or a fracture, or because there was a large filling already in place.

A core builds up the tooth in order to give it substantial structure and stability before placing a crown on it. A core is made from the same materials that a tooth is filled with when decay is removed, thus being amalgam (silver filling) or composite (tooth colored filling). There is a general rule of thumb in deciding if a core is needed. If more than one half of the tooth is missing a core is placed. A dental core gives the tooth stability and builds up the tooth structure.

A post and core are used when the core needs some additional anchorage to the remaining tooth structure. The post takes the place of the nerve and therefore goes into the root of the tooth. Only teeth with completed root canals can have a post. It is important to note that the placement of a post does not make a tooth stronger. A dental post aids in the bonding of the core and the tooth. Dental posts can be made for various materials, including but not limited to gold, titanium, and stainless steel.

Holistic dental treatment does not advocate doing root canals. Holistic dentistry looks as the person as a whole and it is believed that root canals cause the immune system to be affected. Since it is impossible to clean each and every tubule in the root, bacteria grows and toxins get into your body. The tooth is dead and no longer has blood supply. Another controversial issue with root canal treatment is the use of formaldehyde and or creosote to disinfect the inside of treated teeth. Since vapors from these remain inside the tooth, a person with a low functioning immune system may be affected in various ways.

ARE ROOT CANALS NECESSARY?

Bacteria is always present in your mouth and not a problem until there is an infection. There are several types of bacteria known to be in a root canal (Parvimonas, Prevotella, Fusobacterium, Dialister, Streptoccoccus, Treponema). Diseases such as atherosclerosis, Alzheimer's and diabetes have been linked to these bacteria. In the early 1900s Dr. Westin Price began researching the downside of root canals. For the next 25 years he continued to do major studies and experiments around the world on this topic. Dr. Price was the head of research for the National Dental Association, and he had a son who died after receiving a root canal and did not want anyone else to experience the same tragedy. Endocarditis causes the heart valve to become inflamed. His studies concluded that heart disease, as well as circulatory diseases, arthritis and nervous system diseases, can result from a root canal.

One of his experiments involved a wheelchair-bound elderly lady. She also had debilitating arthritis. He advised her to extract her root canaled tooth. Once this was done, the elderly lady had a 100 percent recovery. He took the study further and with this tooth a rabbit was used. The rabbit got the tooth implanted under its skin. The rabbit contracted the same disease as the elderly lady and died ten days later. (The same study was repeated numerous times, and each time a rabbit would exhibit the same symptoms and or disease as the person with the extracted root canal tooth. Yet the person, once the tooth was extracted did have lessening of symptoms and even some recovered completely once RCT was removed.) Studies show that these diseases are transmittable. Autoimmune diseases as well as a link to breast cancer have been found with root canaled teeth. Dr. Price did publish a lot of papers, but the ADA stood by its stance that root canals are safe. Dr. Menig is a Chicago born endodontist who worked in Hollywood CA. He spent almost two years in the early 1990s researching Dr. Price once he came across this information. Dr. Menig published "Root Canal Cover Up" in 1993, and it remains as the authoritative reference on root canals. A cardiologist by the name of Dr. Thomas Levy published a book in 2002 called *The Toxic Tooth* which talks about the hidden infections and root canals. The co-author of this book is Dr. Kulacz who left most of dentistry after learning about these issues. It is said that 100 percent of teeth with root canals have "anaerobic" bacteria. These are more toxic because they do not require oxygen. It is also said that the bacteria seep through into your bloodstream and invade your body. There was a study that showed 98 percent of woman with breast cancer have a root canal tooth on that same side. Dr. Robert Jones works as a researcher at the University of Glasgow. Women with breast cancer were studied over five years. The study had over 300 women participating in it. He found that 93 percent of these women had at least one root canal and most of the cancers were on the same side as their root canal was. The ADA has never published any reports linking root canal treatments to cancer and stands by their claim that RCT are safe. In the United States more than 40,000 root canals are being done daily and over 25 million are done on a yearly basis in the US.

Dr. Weston Price had found in his examination of root canaled teeth toxins called Thio-ethers. These toxins are more potent than the toxin known as botulism.

Dr. Josef Issels was a physician in Germany treating cancer patients. He had found that approximately 97% of his cancer patients had at least one root canaled tooth in their mouth.

Some people do not believe these theories and say that the studies Dr. Price did cannot be duplicated and testing was done in non-sterile conditions.

"Numerous studies in which biopsies were performed on extracted teeth which had been endodontically treated (root canaled) have shown remnants of necrotic debris still in that root canal, meaning that they were not thoroughly cleaned. Microbiological cultures of the surrounding bone showed infection almost 100% of the time. Until anaerobic bacteria are removed, the body's natural defenses are compromised, and those root canal complications can make your health go downhill. The health of your teeth is directly tied to the health of your whole body, and if the anaerobic bacteria are sealed into a root canal tooth, you're liable to have health problems going forward." This as per Dr. Gerry Curatola. He has over 35 years of dental practice experience, is a graduate of NYU Dental School and the founder of Rejuvenation Dentistry.

The Paracelsus Clinic is located in Switzerland and run by Dr. Thomas Ray. He found in 2015 that 147 of his last 150 breast cancer patients had root canals. And they were on the same side as the cancer. This is 98% of the women. There is a biological dental area in this clinic and all cancer patients get all root canaled teeth removed.

White blood cells in the body fight infection. White blood cells travel in the bloodstream but they do not travel to the roots of these teeth, and leave bacteria to flourish and harbor. And the decomposing of the dead tooth tissue continues. However, the American Association of Endodontics claims, "The truth: There is no valid, scientific evidence linking root canal-treated teeth and disease elsewhere in the body. A root canal is a safe and effective procedure. When a severe infection in a tooth requires endodontic treatment, that treatment is designed to eliminate bacteria from the infected root canal, prevent reinfection of the tooth and save the natural tooth."

Sometimes root canals fail and need to be retreated. Some reasons these can fail are canals which were not initially treated, contamination by saliva, new areas of dental decay, and cracks in the tooth. There are also others reasons but these are a few common ones. Sometimes an abscess or bubble forms on the gum near a treated root canal tooth. These bubbles may drain liquid and they may come and go. Antibiotics are recommended in order to help clear the infection. Abscesses can occur on a tooth with a root canal as well as a tooth without one. It is recommended to see an endodontist as well as take antibiotics. You should not pop the abscess. Abscesses occur when there is an infection in your mouth and pus fills up in the abscess. Abscesses can show up on a dental X-ray as well. An abscessed area looks like a black circle at the root of your tooth. The options to treat a failed root canal are to retreat the root canal with a new root canal procedure or to extract the tooth. If the tooth is extracted it is recommended to replace that space with either an implant or a bridge. A bridge is when the adjacent teeth are ground down and have a crown made on each. (A crown is also sometimes called a cap.) The fake tooth that takes the place of the extracted tooth connects to each of the adjacent crowns. This is done with one unit that gets cemented in your mouth. Crowns and bridges are made from porcelain and metal. It is believed that the Romans were the first initiators of both dentures and crowns. Proxybrushes and floss threaders are specific tools used at home to be able to clean underneath and in between these bridges. Implants are made with titanium screws placed in your jawbone. The area fuses together over approximately 6-12 weeks and this implant acts as a tooth root. A crown is secured on top of this with an "abutment" to secure it in place. Implants are the most expensive way to replace a tooth and also the longest lasting way. A dental implant can last a lifetime and have success rates up to 98%.

ROOT CANALS IN PRIMARY TEETH

Sometimes root canals are recommended on primary teeth. This procedure is known as a pulpotomy. A pulpotomy is performed in order to save a primary tooth when the nerve becomes infected. When the pulp chamber becomes infected due to deep area of decay and in order to hold the space until the permanent tooth erupts a pulpotomy is recommended. Pulpotomies are done under local anesthetic.

A pulpectomy is similar to a pulpotomy with one major difference. This difference is in how much of the nerve tissue is removed. In a pulpotomy only the pulp in the crown of the tooth is affected, while in a pulpectomy not only is the crown of the tooth affected but also the root of the tooth. If an abscess is present on the gum tissue, it is recommended that antibiotics be taken first for several days before the procedure is performed. On both the above-mentioned procedures, crowns are placed after completion. On molar teeth a stainless steel crown is used. Crowns used on baby teeth are prefabricated and cemented on. They should remain in place until the tooth is exfoliated and a permanent tooth takes its place. Placing a crown should keep the tooth/teeth strong and resilient and help to keep it bacteria free. There is some controversy in the using of stainless-steel crowns due to the nickel content in them. Nickel has a high allergy rate and these contain up to 12% nickel per crown. Skin breakouts occur with nickel allergies but mouth mucosa does not break out. The average amount of time to do a pulpotomy on a primary molar is 45 minutes whereas the average amount of time to complete a permanent molar root canal is ninety minutes.

Molars are not the only primary teeth that can get pulpotomies. Anterior teeth may need them as well. Some reasons include baby bottle caries, deep decay and or trauma to a tooth or teeth.

As an alternative to a pulpotomy and crown, primary teeth may be extracted. (The same alternative holds true for permanent teeth.) Unlike permanent teeth, baby teeth almost never get bridges placed. Instead space maintainers are used. A space maintainer will hold the place for the permanent tooth to erupt anatomically correct. This aids in the prevention of "malocclusion." Space maintainers are made from metal and are cemented in the mouth adjacent to the space of the missing tooth. These appliances are "passive" and should not cause dental discomfort to the child. Space maintainers are rarely used on adults. The removal of this appliance comes when the permanent tooth is erupting. When a space maintainer is on only one side of the mouth it is known as "unilateral" and when there are space maintainers on both sides of the mouth it is known as "bilateral." Space maintainers are used in both upper and lower arches. If no permanent tooth erupts, the space maintainer usually stays in place until a permanent bridge is made once the child is an adult and stops growing.

When doing a root canal, the canal/canals are first clean out by a tool known as an endodontic file. The canal would be the part in the root that holds the nerve in place. Files are used to help guide and navigate tooth root structure and anatomy. There are several types of endodontic files each with a specific benefit. The following are just a few of the types of files. "Hand Files" are great for tactile sensitivity. "K-type Files" are made from stainless steel alloy and has twisted squares. The "K-flex File" has a cross section that is rhomboid and is more flexible than the "K-type File." "C-type Files" are more rigid than K files and are best used for thin canals and ones with curves. "Nickel-titanium Files" have much more elasticity than over stainless steel files. This elasticity gives them the benefit of less fracture risk. Nickel-titanium files can also be returned to their original shape once heated. Less time is needed in preparation versus stainless and a lower number of files are needed overall.

"Hedstrom Files" are beneficial in root canals being retreated. They are both narrow and very sharp.

Although there are several procedure errors that can occur in a root canal treatment, the most concerning is file separation. This is when a piece of the file breaks inside the canal and according to Wikipedia is the error to be most concerned with. Some reasons for files to break inside a canal include files that are too stiff to maneuver root curvatures. Also, files that are used too much and are weakened, generation of too much torque, defects along the file surfaces, and improper usage by the operator. You may have a "toxic tooth" and yet you may not be experiencing any symptoms.

The newest advance in root canal treatments is the "GentleWave Procedure." The high-tech irrigation process of the GentleWave system "harnesses optimized procedure fluids, vertical flow and broad-spectrum acoustic energies to debride and disinfect the root canal system - even the undetected, un-instrumented spaces - with a minimally invasive protocol that leaves more of the tooth structure intact." It is said to clean canals better than customary procedures used in root canal treatment.

NITROUS OXIDE

Nitrous oxide, better known as "laughing gas" and also called "hippy crack," is sometimes administered when prepping for crowns and doing root canals. The name laughing gas was given to nitrous by a chemist named Humphry Davy. Some side effects of nitrous oxide can include, and are not limited to, dizziness, headache, sweating and shivering. Prolonged exposure can cause memory loss and the depletion of vitamin B-12. When vitamin B-12 depletion is long-term, brain and nerve damage occurs. When breathing in this gas it can take effect immediately. The oxygen/nitrous ratio is controlled on the machine by a professional. It is important to have the proper nitrous to oxygen ratio when using this gas. There are some important contraindications to be aware of. Patients experiencing recent ear nose and or throat infections should not be given nitrous oxide, per Dr. Steven Schwartz DDS. He states that force in the middle ear may increase due to the penetration of the nitrous there. Check with your doctor and dentist, and let them know any medical issues and medications that you are on. Notify the health care professional if you are allergic to latex so a non-latex nasal hood may be substituted.

The FDA's Anesthetic and Life Support Drugs Advisory Committee is investigating data from animal studies suggesting that having to anesthetic agents during the period of high speed brain unfolding produces extended neuronal apoptosis with possible long-term functional results. When contemplating administration of nitrous oxide to pregnant women and to patients under three years of age the benefits and risks of the surgeries should be considered and explained to patients/parents. This committee also advises only one-time exposure to nitrous oxide and a time period of under three hours. The American Dental Association classifies nitrous oxide as a Class C medication while used in pregnancy. This translates as a risk factor for fetal harm. As of April 2019 the ADA states, "It is recommended that pregnant women, both patients and staff, avoid exposure to nitrous oxide." Nitrous oxide is not recommended during trimester one of pregnancy. It is important to know that there are always small amounts of this gas that leak from the nose piece, hoses etc. Since it has no odor or color the patient and staff are unaware of the nitrous oxide in the air.

Would you try to save a dying organ in your body? For example, would you save your gall bladder or appendix if it died? That is what saving a dying tooth is equivalent to. And since the tooth is dead because the nerve is removed, if there is a problem you are unable to feel any pain. Nowhere in your body is it accepted to keep a dead organ or dead tissue. However, a root canal tooth is accepted according to the ADA. The American Academy of Endodontists states that root canals are safe and have been researched. Biological dentists state that root canals may cause health issues such as autoimmune disorders, heart problems and even cancer.

CHAPTER 6
THE 60 SECOND TREATMENT

FLUORIDE

Fluoride toothpaste was launched in 1914. Some composite material does contain fluoride. Fluoride is available in supplements, water, toothpastes, mouthwashes and in a higher concentration at the dental office. Dental grade fluoride comes in a rinse, foam, gel and or varnish. Fluoride, another controversial topic in dentistry, is used in the prevention of dental cavities. Fluoride was discovered in 1901 by a dentist by the name of Frederick McKay. It is known to help prevent dental cavities and it is also known to cause enamel mottling when too much is present in one's body. There is a three-step way in which fluoride works, inhibiting tooth demineralization, enhancing remineralization, and hindering bacterial metabolism.

The American Academy of Pediatrics recommends using fluoride on teeth as soon as they erupt. They also recommend supplemental fluoride vitamins depending on the water concentration, as well as a mouth rinse containing fluoride for those over 6 years old. They also recommend that children start on fluoridated toothpastes right away when teeth erupt and continue to use only toothpaste containing fluoride.

Fluoride varnish, which is applied after a dental cleaning, is covered by Medicaid across the USA now. It is recommended by the AAP that children 6 months old through 16 years old be given fluoride supplementation. Fluoride water levels should be accessed prior to this as to not over-fluoridate them. At home fluoride supplementation is available in either a liquid or a tablet form. It is important not to dispense this one hour prior to or after having milk. Milk and calcium bind and the effect of the fluoride is not as great.

DIFFERENT TYPES OF FLUORIDE

There are several different types of fluoride. Calcium fluoride is found in well water and in soil. Sodium fluoride is the one originally added to drinking water. Sodium fluoride, found in toothpastes, is absorbed by your body and is not naturally occurring. Hydrofluorosilicic acid is the current fluoride in most of today's fluoridated water. This, along with sodium fluoride, is known as toxic. Hydrofluorosilicic contains arsenic and leaches through lead as it travels through pipes.

Silver diamine fluoride is a non-costly topical treatment for dental decay to prevent further spreading. In 2014 the FDA approved the usage of silver diamine fluoride to treat dental hypersensitivity. This material is used off label in the arrest of dental decay in both adults and children, as it has not been approved for this use. Studies show that if decay is not filled that using SDF every six months will be of value. Fluoride varnish is 5% whereas SDF is almost twice the strength (44,800 parts per million), and it is contraindicated to use both on the same day. The reason is because the safety is not known and the fluoride level would be addictive.

While filling a tooth with dental caries gives it back function, using SDF does not do this, nor does it restore the shape. If the teeth are not filled, food impaction may occur, thus leading to a larger area of decay. SDF is not recommended for use in place of a permanent filling, but only to suspend spread of decay. It is recommended that a minimum of two treatments be done to arrest caries. When SDF comes in contact with skin or mouth tissue it causes black staining. The staining will usually resolve in a few days; however, when SDF is placed on tooth surface it will remain black permanently! The black cannot be removed at home or during a professional dental cleaning. Even once a filling is placed it will not disguise the black. When SDF comes in contact with surfaces (floors, walls, countertops, etc.) they will stain black. SDF is colorless and odorless, and looks like water. Contraindications for using SDF include silver allergy, ulcerative gums, and stomatitis (inflammation of the mouth tissues). Stomatitus is a common condition affecting over 200,000 people per year.

CAN FLUORIDE BE HARMFUL TO YOU?

Dental fluorosis is caused from too much fluoride being ingested while teeth are forming and not yet erupted. The damage caused and the white spots and lines that are present on these teeth are permanent. The percentage of children affected with fluorosis has dramatically increased over the years. In 1950 there were 10% of children with fluorosis, 1986 had 23% and in 2004 this jumped to 41%. This study was done on children aged 12-15 and is an astounding 400% escalation. This is due to many more products having fluoride in them (toothpaste, water, food etc.). Dental fluorosis varies from mild to moderate and can be severe. In severe cases the teeth will start to crumble because they are so brittle and porous.

Dr. Hardy Limeback states, "It is illogical to assume that tooth enamel is the only tissue affected by low daily doses of fluoride ingestion." He also stated that fluoride did more harm than good. He was part of a study in 2010 that did not find fluoride effective in dental health. Dr. Hardy Limeback is the head of the University of Toronto's preventive dentistry program.

The late Dr. John Colquhoun said, "Common sense should tell us that if a poison circulating in a child's body can damage the tooth-forming cells, then other harm also is likely." There have been no studies that show ingesting fluoride only goes to the teeth. Paul Connett, PhD is quoted as saying,

"Water fluoridation is a peculiarly American phenomenon. It started at a time when asbestos lined our pipes, lead was added to gasoline, PCBs filled our transformers and DDT was deemed "safe and effective" so that officials felt no qualms spraying kids in school classrooms and seated at picnic tables. One by one all of these chemicals have been banned, but fluoridation remains untouched."

Studies have shown that fluoride increases hip fractures because it builds up in the bones, making them brittle. Masters and Copeland found in a 1999 study that agents in USA fluoride increased the lead uptake and boosted bad behavior in children. Fluoride is a neurotoxin and attracts heavy metals, thus making it more difficult for you to detox yourself of these. There has not been any study or any proof that ingesting fluoride makes it go straight to your teeth. Children under the age of two should not have fluoride whether it be in toothpaste (it says right on the tube), a fluoride tx at the dental office or in digested water.

The American Dental Association stands by their statement that fluoride is safe for use in children and adults.

Forty children got sick at a school arts and craft show in Porgate Michigan in July 1991. The children had vomiting and diarrhea and it was determined that a fluoride injector pump failed. Fluoride levels reached in excess of 90 PPM.

High levels of fluoride were found in the water in Kodiak, Alaska in May 1993, and residents were told not to drink it. One water sample found 22-24 PPM of fluoride.

Research has shown that fluoride may contribute to kidney changes. Mount Sinai Hospital and Mount Sinai School of Medicine released a report in 2019 in *Environmental International* linking fluoride to reduction in kidney and liver function in adolescents. The kidneys take in a higher level of fluoride than other body organs and is the main acception organ of fluoride. Sixty percent of fluoride gets passed in adult urine while only forty five percent excretes in adolescent urine flow. Close to 2000 adolescent participants were a part of this study.

Patients with kidney issues are at risk to have four times as much fluoride absorbed in their bodies than a healthy individual. Fluoride cannot be excreted once kidneys become damaged and thus these patients are at risk for bone damage as well. This has been known fact for over fifty years. Doctors in the 1940s recommended "signs of renal impairment should have radiographic examination of the skeletal system to rule out the existence of fluoride osteosclerosis." At the first congressional hearing on fluoride in 1952, it was determined that a person with kidney trouble should not drink fluoride water. It is also said that "all persons with dental fluorosis and anemia and /or signs renal impairment should have radiographic examinations of the skeletal system to rule out the existence of fluoride osteosclerosis." The National Kidney Foundation has been quoted as saying that there can be an increased risk for kidney patients if they ingest fluoride. Kidney patients must be told the whole story about fluoride. Fluoride is acknowledged to be slightly less toxic than arsenic and slightly more than lead. Dialysis machines do not and cannot use fluoridated water. The National Kidney Foundation did acknowledge that death and/or poisoning to some kidney patients resulted from fluoride leeching through dialysis machine filters.

Kidney stones are not rare and will affect approximately 5% of women and 10% of men by age 70. Kidney stones were found to be almost 5 times higher in areas with fluoride in the 3.5-4.9 ppm (parts per million). This study was published in 2001 in the journal *Urological Research*. Kidney stones are also known as a renal call. Call is the plural for the word calculus, meaning pebble. Kidney stones are known to cause some of the worst pain.

The *Journal of Analytical Chemistry* published a study in 2014 linking fluoridated toothpaste and fluoridated water to an increase in the incidence of urinary stone disease. Urinary stones are made up of magnesium, calcium and fluoride ions. It is a very painful urinary tract disease. Dehydration causes stones to build up in the kidneys or in the bladder.

A rare malignant bone tumor known as osteosarcoma was studied to assess the risk of fluoride exposure. This type of cancer is the fourth most common in the under 25 age group. Osteosarcoma is most prevalent in bone of knees, ankles, shoulders and wrists. These areas have been shown to have a high response to fluoride. The skeleton is host to 99% of the body's fluoride. When children bones are forming the fluoride, uptake is higher. Males show a higher level of fluoride on their bones than females and osteosarcoma is more common in males at a rate of approximately 50%. The study used 10 patients with childhood osteosarcoma and 10 healthy patients. Blood levels were studied, and it was determined that serum fluoride was much higher in the patients with osteosarcoma. There was also found to be a higher level of fluoride in the drinking water of these patients. Therefore, the conclusion was that there is a link between fluoride consumption and osteosarcoma. Before a 2001 study done by Elise Bassin, DDS of Harvard University there was a 1991 study on rats showing the same results - an increase in osteosarcoma with an increase in fluoride intake. The study did not show an increase in female rats or in mice whether male or female. The study was conducted by the U.S. National Toxicology Program. In 2016 Texas did a study and did not find evidence to support a link of fluoridated water and an increase in osteosarcoma. They looked at both male and female.

Fluoride is found in some composite materials.

The amount of maximum recommended daily fluoride recently got lowered.

The amount of fluoride present in the body's teeth and bone is approximately 10,000 times more than fluoride in the body's soft tissues.

Dental fluorosis occurs when the crystalline structure of the tooth is modified during the evolution stage. This alteration is due to too much fluoride intake and the result is white spots or mottled enamel. Once dental fluorosis is present on a tooth you cannot get it off or out of the affected tooth or teeth. Skeletal fluorosis as well as bone fractures, though rare, have been reported from lingering fluoride exposure.

For infants less than six months of age: the review of evidence did not find a preventive effect (reduction in dental caries) with fluoride input in the first six months of life. This is line with the view expressed by the Institute of Medicine (IOM) in 1997 and supported by the American Dental Association's Council on Scientific Affairs statement in 2011 that the protective effect of fluoride in the first six months of life has not been rooted. Studies also show that it is not necessary to increase fluoride during pregnancy as there is no evidence of a reason to do so. A child will show signs of the first teeth erupting at approximately 6 months of age.

The ADA (American Dental Association) tells parents to use low fluoride or non-fluoridated water when making baby formula.

In 2014 the American Dental Association changed its recommendation on infants using fluoride toothpastes. The toothpastes are labeled and say to consult the dentist before using under two years of age. This is because 2-year-olds cannot spit. It is recommended to wait under whatever age the child is able to spit before using a fluoride toothpaste as to minimize a fluorosis risk from ingesting too much. The bloodstream absorbs 93% of ingested fluoride.

The ADA now says a small amount of fluoride toothpaste can be put on a baby's teeth once they erupt and once the child is able to spit (approximately age 3-6) the amount of toothpaste used can then be increased to pea sized. Canadian studies have suggested no child under three have any fluoride and the Canadian Dental Association says no fluoride supplements for this same age group.

Warning labels were required in the 1950s for toothpastes containing fluoride. The labels stated that, in fluoridated water areas, the toothpastes were not to be used. The table on Crest toothpaste read as follows: "Caution: Children under 6 should not use Crest." In 1958 it was no longer required to label toothpastes as such. Present day fluoridated toothpastes contain 1000PPM of fluoride. The USDA mandated toothpastes to carry a warning label if they were sold in the USA. The warning label as of April 7, 1997 was to read: "WARNING: Keep out of reach of children under 6 years of age. If you accidentally swallow more than used for brushing, seek professional help or contact a poison control center immediately." Sixty mg of fluoride can kill a 2-year-old. One hundred twenty mg of fluoride can kill a nine-year-old. One hundred and forty-three mg of fluoride is in a tube of commercial toothpaste.

Some dentists will prescribe a high fluoride toothpaste for their patients. These are not to be used by children and are not meant to be shared. Although side effects do not always happen, there are some to watch for. They include but are not limited to mouth irritation, rash, itching, dizziness and trouble breathing. Medical assistance should be sought if any of these occur.

Manufacturers have stopped making toothpastes with low levels of fluoride. There are many alternatives in toothpaste that do not contain any fluoride and they will be labeled as such. Fluoride toothpastes first came onto the market in the 1950s.

If a young child manages to consume a large amount of high fluoride toothpaste, he or she should be encouraged to vomit and to drink lots of milk to reduce the absorption of fluoride. Urgent medical assistance should be sought. The CDC studied 1700 children ages 3-6 and found 38% were using more toothpaste than recommended. This can contribute to too much fluoride being ingested and has the risk of causing dental fluorosis.

In 2015 the *Journal of Epidemiology and Community Health* published results of a study by the University of Kent. The study revealed that hypothyroidism (underactive thyroid) is 30% higher in people with elevated fluoride exposure. In order to function properly, the thyroid gland needs the proper amount of iodine. Fluoride has been found to displace iodine and thus interfere with levels.

England, where the study took place, has water with 1.0 mg/L and the USA has the upper safe fluoride level marked as 4.0 mg/L.

Another study done in 2015 and published in the *Environmental Health* journal concluded higher fluoride results in higher levels of ADHD. *The Lancet Neurology* March 2014 edition also linked increased fluoride to ADHD.

In 1945 Grand Rapids, Michigan was the first city in the world to introduce fluoride in the drinking water at 1 PPM. In August of 2014, Israel removed fluoride from its water and it is not an option to be allowed to add it in any municipality. Israel first added fluoride in the 1970s and approximately 70% of the country was fluoridated up until this time. The Supreme Court in Israel determined fluoride to be an outdated and no longer widely accepted practice. This was around the same time Portland, Oregon and Wichita, Kansas voted to not have fluoride in their water. Japan does not add fluoride to their water supply.

Western Europe gets its fluoride from salt rather than water. Zurich was the first to launch this practice in 1956. As of 2012 there are eleven countries drinking fluoridated water by over 50% of the people. There are more people drinking fluoridated water in the United States than the rest of the world combined. By the end of 2013 over 4500 medical and dental professionals signed a petition to end water fluoridation. William Marcus, PhD and chief toxicologist for the EPA Water division, was one of these signatures. British Columbia has 11% of its population drinking fluoridated water. They also are prize to the lowest volume of tooth caries in Canada. Some other Canadian regions have as much as 70% of their people drinking fluoridated water yet have a higher incidence of tooth caries. The largest research on decay and fluoride was carried out in 1986-1987.

Children between the ages of 5 and 17 were studied in over 80 places in the country. A total of 39,000 children participated in this study. The study divided the areas into thirds, one third fluoridated, one third non-fluoridated and the remaining third partially fluoridated. The rate of tooth decay proved to be no different in any of the three regions of fluoridation. Native American reservations all have fluoridated water, yet the decay rate is higher than other communities within the United States.

Male infertility and fluoride exposure were studied using mice in 2013. This study was published in the *Journal Archives of Toxicology. The* results show that fluoride lowered fertility in the mice.

Male testosterone levels are reduced with higher levels of fluoride according to five studies done in China, India, Mexico and Russia (Hao 2010, Ortiz 2003, Susheela 1996, Michael 1996, Tokar 1977)

The U.S. National Institutes of Health along with The U.S. Environmental Protection Agency and the U.S. National Institute of Environmental Health Sciences funded studies on fluoride safety and pregnancy. These studies were the first to show a correlation between fetus -fluoride exposure and reduced IQ. The urine of pregnant women was measured to see how much fluoride was present. There was a 12-year study published in 2017 and the largest study was done with 512 mother-child in Paris and that was published in 2019.

It has been studied and shown by the World Health Organization that countries in Europe without fluoridated water do not have a higher incidence of tooth decay than countries that do fluoridate their water.

The Fluoride Action Network says "drinking water fluoridation actually involves adding a concoction of chemicals - sodium fluoride, sodium fluorosilicate, and hydrofluorosilicic acid - that are in fact unpurified waste products from industry and mining, which in some cases are contaminated with other toxic pollutants, such as arsenic."

Hydrofluorosilicic acid is highly corrosive and is also associated with leaching lead from lead pipes, resulting in higher exposure to lead, another toxic drinking water contaminant.

The EPA considers fluoride to be toxic waste. Fluoride is an aluminum waste product. Iron and copper factories poisoned people and plants with fluoride when it was airborne on purpose in the 1850s. Fluoride could be disposed of legally but in small amounts only. It was sold to rat poison and insecticide manufactures. In a memorable moment in 1939, the first public motion that the U.S. should fluoridate its water supplies was made, not by a doctor or dentist, but by Cox, an industry scientist engaged in employment by a company vulnerable by fluoride damage claims. Almost overnight…"the popular image of fluoride - which at the time was being widely sold as rat and bug poison - became that of a beneficial provider of gleaming smiles, absolutely safe, and good for children, bestowed by a benevolent paternal government. Its opponents were permanently engraved on the public mind as crackpots and right-wing loonies. A lot of people who were originally pro fluoridation changed their minds after seeing the evidence."

The American Dental Association stated in 1988 that a reduction of tooth decay was 40-60% with fluoride and later changed the numbers to be 18-25% reduction. The EPA raised the fluoride standard level from 2.4 to 4PPM in 1986.

A National Institute for Dental research report has said, "It is likely that if caries in children remain at low levels or decline further, the necessity of continuing the current variety and extent of fluoride-based prevention programs will be questioned."

Fluoride is not only found in water to which it is added. Fluoride is contained in many foods as well. The *Journal of Clinical Pediatric Dentistry* tested juices and 42% were found to have over 1PPM of fluoride. Some grape juice was tested at up to 6.8 PPM of added fluoride. The belief is that the grapes have fluoride-containing insecticide.

Fluoride levels are increased when cooking foods. Raw peas have 12 micrograms of fluoride yet once fluoridated water is used to cook them, 1500 micrograms of fluoride is present.

The Mohawk Indians filed a lawsuit in 1960 against the Aluminum Company of America (Alcoa) and Reynolds Metals Company. The out-of-court settlement was reached at $650,000 for their cows. Industrial fluoride was toxic to their community. "Cows crawled around the pasture on their bellies, inching along like giant snails. So, crippled they could not stand up, this was the only way they could graze. Some died kneeling, after giving birth to stunted calves. Others kept on crawling until, no longer able to chew because their teeth had crumbled down to the nerves, they began to starve…"

The Medical Tribune on February 22,1990 said this after an NTP cancer by fluoride study: "It is difficult to see how the EPA can fail to regulate fluoride as a carcinogen in light of what NTP has found. Osteosarcomas are an extremely unusual result in rat carcinogenity tests. Toxicologists tell me that the only other substance that has produced this is radium… The fact that this is a highly atypical form of cancer implicates fluoride as the cause. Also, the osteosarcomas appeared to be dose-related, and did not occur in controls, making it a clean study."

The ADA took the stance that the animals were ingesting high levels of fluoridation in this study. James Huff, the director of the U.S. National Institute of Environmental Health Sciences, answered by saying, "The reason these animals got a few osteosarcomas was because they were given fluoride… Bone is the target organ for fluoride." William Marcus is a toxicologist who added "fluoride is a carcinogen by any standard we use. I believe EPA should act immediately to protect the public, not just on the cancer data, but on the evidence of bone fractures, arthritis, mutagenicity, and other effects."

It was found by The New Jersey Department of Health that young men have a three times higher chance of getting bone cancer in highly fluoridated water areas.

San Francisco saw a 400% increase in cancer once their water became fluoridated.

The EPA does not mandate fluoride addition to water; it is an individual state mandate.

The FDA proposes (April 2019) the allowed level of fluoride in bottled water be lowered to 0.7 mg/L.

NJ is only second to Hawaii in the lowest fluoride in water amounts. One single water utility is the supplier for multiple municipalities in NJ and all municipalities on the water line must agree to fluoridate in order for this to occur. However, legislation is pending to possibly make fluoridation mandatory.

Fluoride is present in approximately half of all prescription drugs. Fluoride is said to affect their magnesium in your body. It also affects the production of glutathione on the body.

Researchers from Harvard University studied IQ scores of children. The study was done in 2013, comparing children in high areas of water fluoridation to children in low fluoridated areas. The results were that the children in the high fluoridated areas had an IQ which was significantly lower than those in low fluoride zones. This was not the only study to have those results.

The *Journal of Epidemiology and Community Health* published a study done in 2015 by the University of Kent researchers. This study found that "people exposed to fluoride in their drinking water were 30 percent more likely to be diagnosed with hypothyroidism." Iodine is said to be displaced by fluoride. More than 3 million people a year are diagnosed with hypothyroidism. It is said to be "very common" in adults over 19 years of age and "common" in teens age 14-18.

Some believe that fluoride, FL2, and neurotoxin are all synonyms. And some people believe it is the best cavity prevention. Almost 50 articles on fluoride toxicity are located at The National Medical Library.

CHAPTER 7
MERCURY RISING

AMALGAM RESTORATIONS

Another ongoing controversial topic in dentistry is amalgam. Amalgam restorations are also known as silver or mercury fillings. These fillings are a mixture of several materials including silver, mercury, copper and possibly zinc palladium. Mercury makes up approximately one half of this combination of metals. Although composite fillings are popular now, amalgam is stronger and holds up better to wear and tear. The usage of amalgam began over 150 years ago. In 2009 the FDA studied amalgam due to concerns of mercury and deemed it a safe material to be used in people over the age of 6.

The official FDA website states, "The developing neurological systems in fetuses and young children may be more sensitive to the neurotoxic effects of mercury vapor." Mercury does release vapors which when inhaled are absorbed by the lungs. When mercury is pure, it is in liquid form. Mercury is known to bioaccumulate in body organs and tissues. Bioaccumulation happens because a substance is absorbed faster than it can be excreted. In studies performed on healthy individuals it was found that being exposed to mercury vapor from amalgam fillings does bioaccumulate in such areas as the kidneys and the brain. The main area of absorption from vapors occurs in the lungs. Elemental mercury releases vapors and is what's found in amalgam fillings. Methylmercury, an organic mercury, is what is found in fish. This type of mercury gets absorbed in your digestive tract. Since removal of amalgam fillings exposes you to mercury vapors, the FDA recommends you leave them in your mouth unless you are having an allergic reaction to them. The amount of mercury released from amalgam has not been determined, although many studies have been done.

It used to be thought that no mercury was released but that theory has been disproven. The FDA advises pregnant women not to get amalgam fillings as mercury can cross the placenta. Too much mercury (of any type) can result in mercury toxicity. Testing for this can be done by a hair sample, urine sample or a blood draw. Symptoms of mercury toxicity include and are not limited to tremors, insomnia, headache, muscle atrophy, and twitching. When a tooth gets an amalgam filling, or one is removed in a dental office, an amalgam trap should be present. It is required by the Environmental Protection Agency that at least 95 % of the amalgam is captured.

When amalgam is captured, the chance of leakage into the sewer system is reduced. Used amalgam capsules are to be recycled and are not to be disposed of in biohazard waste receptacles. Scrap amalgam as well as extracted teeth with amalgam need to be recycled. The reason amalgam is not meant for biohazard waste is that biohazard waste gets incinerated. If amalgam gets incinerated, it releases toxic vapors into the environment.

Amalgam is not only a controversial issue in the USA. Across the world amalgam presents with negativity. Sweden has banned the usage of amalgam due to health concerns. In Norway and Denmark amalgam is banned because of the environmental disposal factors. Canada and the USA have toxicity warnings in effect. The Canadian Dental Association states on their website that mercury does in fact cross the placenta.

The USA started using amalgam fillings in the 1830s and it was thought to be an inferior material. Every member of the American Society of Dental Surgeons was made to sign a document ensuring they would not use it. The usage of amalgam was labeled malpractice. The American Dental Association was formed in 1859, three years after the ASDS ended, and the ADA took the amalgam ban away. The FDA did set 0.4 micrograms intake for every kilogram of body weight as acceptable daily. Studies have shown that with mercury leakage from chewing, grinding, etc. the average person is getting

3-17 micrograms per day or up to 50% more than the accepted amount per the FDA.

Pharmaceutical products have safety testing different than amalgam, as the FDA does not regulate amalgam. In the United States, amalgam is not related as a material by the FDA, but as a prosthetic device. Mercury was classified as class 1 risk (the least risky) until 2009. In 2009 amalgam became a class 11 risk material and needed to have a warning label inside. This warning states, "Dental amalgam has been demonstrated to be an effective restorative material that has benefits in terms of strength, marginal integrity, suitability for large occlusal surfaces, and durability. Dental amalgam also releases low levels of mercury vapor, a chemical that at high exposure levels is well-documented to cause neurological and renal adverse health effects."

Hal Huggins lost his dental license due to "deceptive yet seductive advertising" when he began advocating for dental amalgam removal in the 1970s. He claimed the leakage of mercury was causing such things as MS, lupus, leukemia, etc. There are a group of dentists trying to get legislation to ban the usage of amalgam fillings for everyone. Dr. Huggins is credited with taking blood samples from patients before and after removal of amalgam restorations. He found blood levels were compromised until the removal of mercury from the patient's mouth.

The phrase "Mad as a Hatter" dates back to the 1700s and 1800s. Felt hats worn in England were made with trace amounts of mercury. Mercury poisoning became a prevalent issue amongst many of the hat factory workers. The applied meaning was that a person was insane.

Composite or tooth colored or white fillings are the popular option to dental amalgam restorations. Intrinsic toxic issues are a huge concern, however.

Dental composites start out as a soft material then get light "cured" and harden in the mouth. They then get their final shaping and smoothness and there isn't any downtime. They do not last as long as a dental amalgam would, which is of concern to some. BPA (Bisphenol A) is part of the composite makeup. BPA is a chemical that comes with controversy. BPA is thought to mimic estrogen effects in the human body. Responsible composite manufacturers claim that there is no unreacted BPA in dental resins, and that it takes high temperatures - several hundred degrees - to liberate free BPA.

According to studies done on animals, BPA increases cancer risks. Although studies conducted on animals did not yield any conclusive results, experts feel BPA brings on hormonal effects. These effects can affect the developing fetus and infant. The National Toxicology Program at the FDA has voiced concerns that BPA exposure in infants and young children probably will affect the brain. Humans come in contact with BPA in plastic and canned foods and drinks. No human studies have been done to test the effects of BPA. The US FDA does not believe that BPA is a public health concern, and maintains that composite resins containing Bisphenol-A can be safely used.

Some disadvantages to using composite fillings over amalgam fillings are: they are more costly than amalgam, they take longer to do, they will stain over time and they can't withstand forces as great as amalgam when it comes to chewing.

DISEASES LINKED TO MERCURY

Mercury is considered toxic waste. Mercury goes from the tooth directly into the bloodstream, thus exposing unborn babies to mercury while in the womb. Calomel is a powder containing mercury. It was given to babies in the 1940s for teething pain. This subsequently caused what was known as pink disease. Pink disease caused both cognitive and psychiatric disorders. Thimerosal was used in vaccines for over 50 years and was removed from most of them in 2001. Mercurochrome was banned by the FDA in 1998 after it was once considered safe. It was banned after determining the high mercury content. Amalgam fillings (silver fillings) are still used in the USA, yet banned from most of Europe due to too much mercury. Many restrictions are placed over mercury fillings in both Finland and Japan. Autopsies show the amount of mercury in a body is directly linked to how many fillings are in the mouth.

According to the *Independent*, this is what the FDA stated approximately ten years ago "After years of insisting the fillings are safe, the US government's Food and Drug Administration (FDA) has issued a health warning about them. It represents a landmark victory for campaigners, who say the fillings are responsible for a range of ailments, including heart conditions and Alzheimer's disease. Earlier this month, in an unprecedented U-turn, the FDA dropped much of its reassuring language on the fillings from its website, substituting: "Dental amalgams contain mercury, which may have neurotoxic effects on the nervous systems of developing children and fetuses." It adds that when amalgam fillings are "placed in teeth or removed they release mercury vapor", and that the same thing happens when chewing. The FDA is now reviewing its rules and may end up restricting or banning the use of the metal ".

On July 28, 2009 the FDA stated "the mercury used in dental amalgam fillings is not at a level high enough to cause harm in patients, according to the FDA, which today issued its final regulation on the controversial tooth filling material. However, the agency tightened its controls on mercury fillings, classifying the encapsulated amalgams now commonly sold to dentists as Class II devices, deemed a moderate risk, instead of the lower class I devices." Also, according to the FDA, the vapor from the mercury is released when chewing, as well as when the mercury is removed.

The American Dental Association was in agreement with the FDA in not placing restrictions on dental amalgam use.

Between the years 1989–2009, 141 complaints of adverse reactions from amalgam were filed with the FDA.

The *International Journal of Dentistry* stated that mercury can leak from amalgam filling in the form of a vapor. They also say it is rare to have an allergic reaction, and systemic disease and/or toxicology is not caused from mercury vapors.

In November 2019, Andrew Cuomo, Governor of New York, consented legislation which bans installing floors containing mercury in schools there. This legislation will begin in 2020. There is a ban in place now that also prohibits the existing flooring being covered up. Limits will be in place immediately as far as mercury exposure for both students and employees. This law is set for public and private schools as well as elementary and secondary schools. Flooring installed from 1960-1990 often contained mercury. This is especially evident in the gymnasium rubber floorings. Mercury vapors can be emitted through these floorings, and can cause side effects. According to the new law, all flooring containing mercury must be removed before the new floors can be installed, starting in 2021.

Even though it is known that, given enough mercury, there is human toxicity, most researchers agree that mercury-based fillings do not cause mercury poisoning in people. Breathing a large quantity of metallic mercury can cause poisoning. Some researchers believe the amount emitted from amalgam fillings is not a large enough amount to cause any issues. Metallic mercury travels through the bloodstream to various organs quickly, but the most dangerous and concerning is the brain.

Without mercury there is no Alzheimer's Disease. A study published in the *Journal of Alzheimer's Disease* November 2010 states, "New research by Northeastern University professor Richard Deth and academic colleagues in Germany suggests that long-term exposure to mercury may produce Alzheimer's - like symptoms in people. Deth also discovered a probable biological mechanism through which mercury can destroy neurological brain function in humans." There were 100 studies involving cells, animals as well as humans. Animals in the study exposed to mercury showed changes pathologically mimicking Alzheimer's Disease. Some symptoms included confusion and memory loss. Data cannot link this one hundred percent to humans, but data shows a need to be cautious on mercury exposure. Professor Deth stated, "Mercury is clearly contributing to neurological problems, whose rate is increasing in parallel with rising levels of mercury. It seems that the two are tied together." It was found by Professor Deth that selenium efficacy was impaired when exposed to mercury, thus causing an impairment of cognitive function. Selenium is an antioxidant which helps keep the brain healthy by suppressing damaging chemical reaction in humans. Mercury and selenium bind together, lowering the number of antioxidants available. Nerves stop functioning normally, cognitive impairment sets in and cells die. "Does Inorganic Mercury play a Role in Alzheimer's Disease?" is a paper co-authored by Professor Deth. Other colleagues included on this paper are from the Institute of Transcultural Health Studies, located at the European University Vladrina, the European Office of the Samueli Institute, and the Department of Environmental and Integrative Medicine, Konstanz, all in Germany.

Fourteen million people are projected to have Alzheimer's Disease by the year 2050. And dementia will affect 130 million people by this same year. Alzheimer's is non-reversible, and it progresses. In the year 2018 it was estimated that 5.7 million people had a diagnosis of Alzheimer's Disease. Numerous studies and reports have been done linking or not linking dental amalgams and Alzheimer's Disease. *The Lancet* did a study in 1999 which said that dental amalgams, although releasing a vapor, do not reach the brain. Dementia to date has over 100 forms. Alzheimer's makes up at least one half of the cases.

PRECAUTIONS AND REMOVAL PROCESS OF MERCURY FILLINGS

In June 2001, *Consumers for Dental Choice* sued both the American Dental Association and the California Dental Association, stating that patients are purposely deceived when amalgam fillings, which contain about 50% mercury, also called silver fillings. The American Dental Association takes the stance of mercury is safe and they aren't hiding amalgam contains mercury. Boyd Haley, professor and chairman of the department of chemistry at the University of Kentucky, has testified on dental mercury danger before Congress. "They place this stuff in people's mouths and it's toxic before it goes in, and it's toxic when it is placed on your tooth, so how does it suddenly become safe?"

WebMD says some dentists told them they do not warn patients of dental mercury vapor because they do not think it is harmful to the patient. Such daily things as eating drinking hot liquids and brushing causes vapor to escape.

In 2009 The World Health Organization suggested phasing out mercury in dentistry.

Maryland State Dental Board had five dentists with a lawsuit. Their suit states the dental board "gag rules keep dentists from being able to openly discuss the mercury to their patients." Bill DeLong DDS is dentist in that lawsuit. He told WebMD that he has been brought before his state dental board twice for talking to patients about the safety precautions he uses in his office— including a mercury vapor detector — when removing fillings. He continues by stating, "I had complaints ...about the fact that I discuss that with patients, and in both instances, they tried to either confiscate my instruments or get me to not discuss anything with my patients unless they bring it up first."

Dr. Boyd Haley chairs the Chemistry Department at University of Kentucky. He is an expert on mercury and contends that mercury is a neurotoxicant which can cause many diseases.

Removing mercury fillings has the risk of contaminating water as mercury gets into the water supply. According to the World Health Organization (WHO), over one half (53%) of environmental mercury emissions is from amalgam and laboratory accessories. The EPA recommends that dentists use amalgam separators to catch and hold excess amalgam waste, to decrease the release of mercury into the sewer system.

The use of dental amalgam was prohibited in Scandinavian countries as of 2008, for the betterment of environmental and health. Participants in Sweden with chronic fatigue type symptoms had amalgam fillings removed. Seventy-eight percent of these participants reported increased health.

In 2001, the US National Health and Nutrition Examination surveyed 31,000 adults and found that the number of dental fillings correlated to the incidence of cancer, mental conditions, thyroid conditions, neurological issues (including MS), diseases of the respiratory system, and diseases of the eye. However, the United States, FDA and various Supreme Court justices determined that the correlations do not sufficiently demonstrate causation.

Mercury vapor is at its highest when the amalgam is placed or removed from a tooth.

When replacing and or removing an amalgam restoration it is important that safety measures are in place. A rubber dam should be placed on the tooth being worked on. This will reduce the vapors in the environment and will confine the specific tooth. It also keeps mercury dust and pieces from coming in contact with dental tissues. If amalgam hits the side of the tongue it is the quickest route of absorption. Suction should be close to the tooth and high-speed suction is the best choice. Make sure the patient breathes through their nose, not their mouth. Patients should have protective plastic gear underneath the dental bib. Eyes should be protected with goggles as to keep particles from entering. Dental personnel are also urged to wear protective eye gear, masks, disposable gloves and disposable gowns. It has been demonstrated that these particles can be spread from the patient's mouth to the hands, arms, face, chest, and other parts of the dental worker's and patient's anatomy.

The International Academy of Oral Medicine and as Toxicology is a scientific, biological dental organization. It is a global network of dentists, health professionals, and scientists who research the biocompatibility of dental products, including the risks of mercury fillings, fluoride, root canals, and jawbone osteonecrosis. The "IAOMT was founded in 1984 and is non-profit. They have served as expert witnesses through their research and studies for US Congress, US FDA, Health Canada as well as in the Philippines and in Europe.

OSHA (Occupational Safety and Health Act) states that "higher levels of mercury exposure can result in permanent nervous system and kidney damage. When handling amalgam and amalgam waste, dentists could be exposed to mercury in amounts that exceed federal safety standards. Removal of dental amalgams one instance where this could be the case. OSHA therefore requires these employees wear respiratory protection. This requirement is in place because some amounts of mercury can be released when working with amalgam fillings. No, this amount in itself is not enough to harm the dentist, either. The concern, though, is that the dentist is performing these tasks often and repeatedly throughout the day, day after day."

On July 14, 2017 a rule went into effect requiring general dentists to have an amalgam separator in place. This would keep amalgam from getting into the air and water. July 14, 2020 is the compliance date for dentists to have these. This requirement is for dental offices which release their wastewater into a POTW- Publicly Owned Treatment Work. Existing office not exempt from the rule must install a compliant separator no later than July 14,2020; newly constructed or purchased offices must immediately install a separator and submit a one - time compliance report within 90 days of taking ownership.

Offices which are exempt from having the amalgam separators include offices that exclusively practice at least one of these specialties: oral pathology, oral and maxillofacial radiology, oral and maxillofacial surgery, orthodontics, periodontics, and prosthodontics, as well as mobile dental units or offices that discharge wastewater into a private septic system. Offices that do not place amalgam restorations are also exempt. Offices that have amalgam separators in place currently can continue with those. However, the timeline is until the lifetime of the unit is over or until July 14, 2027, whichever date comes first.

More information on amalgam separators and the rule are available on the ADA website.

There are regulations state federal and local which dentists must comply with in regard to mercury disposal. These regulations also govern the proper handling of the mercury and cleaning of the room in which the mercury was removed.

CHAPTER 8
ONE OF THESE THINGS JUST DOESN'T BELONG

WHY IS THAT IN YOUR MOUTH?

Aphthous ulcers are also known as canker sores. These are very common, small white and shallow sores found inside the mouth. They are not contagious and will last approximately 10 days. Most minor aphthous ulcers are white and oval in shape with a reddened border and require no medication. Since they are somewhat sore it may cause difficulty eating or drinking certain foods and liquids. Some possible causes include stress, vitamin deficiency and poor fitting dentures. Aphthous ulcers seem to be more common in females than males, and approximately 20% of both male and females do get recurrent ulcers.

Sodium laureth sulfate (SLES) is an ingredient in certain toothpastes. It is thought this ingredient may trigger an aphthous ulcer breakout in some. SLES is different than sodium lauryl sulfate (SLS) in that SLES is gentler. SLES also has the ability to foam more. The American Cancer Society does not list SLES as a cancer-causing agent. The National Institute for Health does find that using SLS produces irritation in those who suffer from apthous ulcers. *Forbes* says that repeated use can cause SLS allergies. The *Wall Street Journal* has found that eczema or dermatitis sufferers can have a more intense allergic reaction with SLS. The Centers for Disease Control cautions that repeated use of SLS can cause dermatitis and that irritation from powder form even short term can occur. They also caution that toxins can be emitted if SLS is burned and at a high temperature SLS is combustible. According to the CDC, SLS is "toxic to fresh-water organisms" but the NIH "qualifies that the surfactant is 99 percent environmentally friendly." The National Institute for Occupational Safety and Health says kidneys, liver and the central nervous system can all be affected negatively.

When SLS is not diluted and ingested symptoms such as nausea, diarrhea and vomiting can arise and mercola.com has found SLS and SLES to be a possible carcinogenic to humans. It is important to note that SLS is not used without dilution in toothpastes and other products.

Only about 15% of toothpastes on the market do not contain SLS. Although your bloodstream can absorb SLS, it is not on the list of neurotoxins.

Fluoride uptake is diminished by the usage of SLS and SLS can increase sensitivity issues in the mouth.

Herpes cold sores are also known as fever blisters and are not aptheous ulcers. Herpes cold sores are contagious and caused by a virus. Incubation period averages 4 days and ranges from 2-12 days. Before a herpes breakout tingling or itching can be felt at the site. Blisters erupt and then crust over. Herpes Simplex virus one as it is otherwise known affects approximately 67% of the population throughout the world. On average the sores last 7-14 days and healing time may be speeded up with use of an antiviral agent.

The HSV lies dormant in the nerve ganglion until a breakout gets triggered. Some factors that bring on breakouts include, but are not limited to, stress, fevers, and trauma. Breakouts can also come without any triggering factors. Usually an HSV breakout re-occurs in the same area.

Herpes Whitlow is when fingers break out with a herpes sore(s). Herpes Whitlow is common for healthcare providers who use their hands in people's mouths. Even though gloves are used as barrier protection, a herpes virus can enter the finger(s).

Candida is a yeast-caused fungal infection. Candida survives in various places in the body, including the mouth. When a candida infection is present in the mouth it is called thrush or oral thrush. Candida Albicans is the most common type of candida. Thrush is harmless and usually goes away on its own quickly. Thrush is seen quite often in infants as well as people with compromised immune systems. People suffering from asthma who need steroid sprays are at risk to develop a thrush infection. Using antibiotics can also bring on a thrush outbreak. Smokers have a higher risk of getting , as well as denture wearers when dentures are ill-fitting. And, stress is a cause of thrush as well as many oral conditions. The telltale signs of thrush include a white area on gum tissues, cheeks, tonsils, throat, etc. This white area is raised a little. Sometimes there is pain and sometimes no pain is felt. There may or may not be bleeding the area gets abraded. Yeast is present in the body and is usually kept under control. When this control is escalated the thrush appears. Sometimes an antifungal will be prescribed by the dentist for treatment of thrush. Decreasing your intake of sugar and yeast can be a preventative measure.

INGREDIENTS IN TOOTHPASTE

Here are some ingredients in toothpaste that are controversial for some people. Triclosan is a pesticide that was banned from soap by the FDA in 2016. However after the ban one toothpaste still had triclosan in it. (This specific toothpaste got revamped in 2019 and the triclosan ingredient removed.) Triclosan was marketed as an antibacterial and preventer of plaque and gingivitis. Even if you do not swallow toothpaste, the effects can be absorbed by gingival tissues. Toothbrushes hold on to chemicals in toothpastes, even if you change your toothpaste of choice. Some concerns of triclosan include but are not limited to cancer, deformed bones, liver problems and heart muscle function that becomes weakened. The FDA does say triclosan is safe in toothpaste, even though they banned it from other over the counter items. *Environmental Science & Technology* published an article on triclosan and toothbrush retention October 2017. The recommended brushing habit of twice a day for two minutes each time was simulated over a ninety day time period. Six toothpastes and 22 toothbrushes were used in this study. More than 33% of the brushes had accumulated 7-12.5% times more triclosan than amounts in one brushing.. Even after changing toothpastes to non-triclosan, the toothbrushes held onto the triclosan ingredient for approximately 14 days. It is also thought that triclosan gets released in the air when disposed of on a toothbrush. Triclosan has been found in wastewater and found to be toxic to aquatic life.

Saccharin is also found in some toothpastes. It is a lab-produced sweetener that is over 300 times sweeter than sugar. In the 1970s clinical studies linked saccharin to cancer in rats and almost 50 years later saccharin is still used in foods and products sold for hygiene. The sole purpose of adding sodium saccharin to toothpaste is flavor enhancement. No benefit for the health of the oral cavity has been found.

Aspartame is sweeter than sugar by about 200% and is a common sugar substitute. Aspartame has been known to metabolize inside your body as both a poisonous wood alcohol and formaldehyde. Formaldehydes are used as embalming fluids. Aspartame has been linked to numerous side effects and diseases. Some of these include nausea, dizziness, seizures, depression and memory loss. Alzheimer's, diabetes and fibromyalgia have also been linked to aspartame consumption.

Sorbitol is another flavor enhancement. Unlike saccharin or aspartame, sorbitol is not as sweet as table sugar and is usually combined with another sweetener. Sorbitol also has not been found to enhance oral health and if used in large amounts can have effects similar to laxatives.

Sodium Lauryl Sulfate is the ingredient which produces a foaming effect in toothpastes. One interesting fact about SLS is that this was first used as a floor cleaner. According to The American Cancer Society it is not a cancer causing agent, but SLS is a known irritant. The National Institute of Health reports that mouth sores and stomatitis symptoms may be enhanced with the use of SLS. the Wall street Journal says SLS can irritate skin and The Center for Disease Control has found that dermatitis can occur from long-term usage.

Carrageenan can be found in natural toothpastes as well as conventional ones. It is a thickening agent and has been possibly linked to tumors of the colon and inflammation of the intestine.

Parabens are commonly added to toothpaste and cosmetics in order to prolong shelf-life. Due to their chemical make-up , they have the ability to mimic estrogen. WebMD cites a study done in October 2015 claiming even small amounts of parabens can start the growth of certain cancerous cells. Parabens have restrictions overseas and Europe has a 100% ban on five parabens. As of September 2019 the FDA stands by their thinking that health is not endangered from cosmetically used parabens.

Carrageenan is an additive in some toothpaste as a thickener. Intestinal inflammation and ulcers are potential side effects. The soft tissues in the oral cavity absorb carrageenan so swallowing is not needed in order to experience side effects.

DEA is a foaming agent in toothpaste. Nitrosamines are chemical compounds, most of which are carcinogenic. They are used in the manufacture of cosmetics, pesticides, tobacco products and in most rubber products like balloons and condoms. When DEA interacts with some toothpaste ingredients, nitrosamines are formed.

Preservatives which release formaldehyde are also found in some toothpastes. The US doesn't have strict restrictions like Europe and Canada. When formaldehyde is released, the mucosal tissues absorb it.

Some toothpastes contain GMOs. Certified organic toothpastes and non-GMO verified pastes do not contain items such as these.

Propylene glycol and PEGs (polyethylene glycol) assist other ingredients in penetrating skin. PEGs are notoriously contaminated with 1.4-dioxane (a carcinogen). Propylene glycol is used in toothpastes for smoothing the texture.

Artificial colors are used in some toothpastes for coloring and not a necessary ingredient. Dyes such as D&C Red 30, FD&C Blue 1 and D&C Yellow 10 can build up over prolonged use and affect organs.

CAVITATIONS

Sometimes getting a tooth extracted doesn't end your problem, but starts a "HOLE" new one. A cavitation is a cavity in your bone. This usually happens after an extraction when the bone does not heal correctly. Osteonecrosis is a space of dead bone where it never filled in correctly. When the periodontal ligament (tissues which are attached to the bone) is left behind during/after an extraction the risk of cavitation is present. Experts speculate that this incomplete healing occurs because the bone cells on both sides of the extraction site sense the presence of the periodontal membrane and "think" the tooth is still there.

Bacteria breed and multiply inside cavitation spaces and cause health issues that can become chronic. Almost one half of cavitations are found where wisdom teeth have been removed. Cavitations are found using a special type of X-ray machine and will not typically be diagnosed on a standard X-ray.

Cavitations are treated by surgically cleaning the area and taking out the diseased bone.

Other reasons for cavitation can include insufficient circulation, injury, steroid usage, and clotting issues, to name a few.

LET'S KEEP IT CLEAN

Per the American Dental Association, there is a "cosmetic mouthwash" and there is a "therapeutic mouthwash." Also, according to the ADA, they are used for different reasons. Cosmetic mouthwashes are solely for breath freshening whereas therapeutic mouthwashes have different ingredients to serve individual issues.

Bad breath is said to be lowered with cetylpyridinum chloride (CPC). CPC is also found in some toothpastes and lozenges. It has been shown to kill bacteria and inhibit plaque formation. Some pesticides also contain CPC in their list of ingredients. A class action suit was filed by a group of people whose teeth turned brown as a result of CPC in mouthwash. This resulted in a disclaimer on the mouthwash which states, "In some cases, antimicrobial rinses may cause surface staining to teeth." There was one study conducted which resulted in teeth not becoming stained with brown color. It has also been discovered that 3% of people using CPC have staining on their teeth. One company has said staining is a good sign and shows death of the bacteria. All CPC-based oral hygiene products have been approved by the American Dental Association.

The next ingredient in therapeutic mouthwash is essential oils. The purpose of these is plaque reduction. Some popular essentials oils for dental reasons are as follows and are not limited to these oils. Clove oil is an infection fighter and bacteria inhibitor. Clove is also excellent for a toothache. Thyme is a taste enhancer with roots in the mint family. Tea tree oil can help lower inflammation and red gums. Peppermint oil also helps in the reduction of bacteria. In one 2015 study, lemongrass oil was found to be more effective than traditional chlorehexidine mouthwash at reducing plaque and gingivitis levels. To use a lemongrass mouthwash: Dilute two to three drops of lemongrass essential oil in a cup of water. Swish the solution in your mouth for up to 30 seconds.

Fluoride is used in these as well. (See Chapter titled "The Sixty Second Treatment" to learn more on fluoride.) Late in 2010, the FDA warned three mouthwash manufacturers to stop suggesting that their products that have fluoride as the main ingredient would prevent gum disease and remove dental plaque, the sticky biofilm of bacteria and other substances that collects on teeth above and below the gumline.

Peroxide is present in mouthwash to make teeth whiter. Hydrogen peroxide is very good for the health of your gums. Rinse with hydrogen peroxide for about a minute then spit. Do not ingest it. Peroxide foams from the releasing of oxygen and this is what cleans the mouth. Mixing hydrogen peroxide with baking soda and salt is known as Keyes Technique and is excellent for gum health. Mix the two together into a paste. Use on the gums and if the taste bothers you add essential oils and/or mouthwash. The Keyes technique is named after Paul H. Keyes. He died at the age of 99 on February 7, 2017. The Keyes technique was nicknamed the "Salt and Soda" method. Dr. Keyes also played a role in the development of home use daily fluoride gel and the fluoride delivering custom trays. Make sure to follow instructions as to if the peroxide you are using needs to be diluted or not.

The invention of dental floss is said to be that of New Orleans dentist Levi Spear Parmly in 1815. In 1882 unwaxed dental floss was marketed. The first patent was given in 1898 to floss made with silk such as the silk in stitches. Waxed dental floss was developed in the 1940s with silk replacing nylon. Nylon was introduced by Charles C. Bass. He explained there was better durability with nylon and it had more stretch to it. In the 1950s dental tape made its debut.

Flossing should be done on a daily basis for optimal oral health. Begin by taking a piece approximately 18" long. Using waxed or unwaxed is personal preference. Wrap the floss around your middle fingers until there is space to hold a piece about an inch with your index fingers and thumbs. See saw the floss in between each tooth gently. Once it reaches the gumline, shape it like a "C" and go up and down on the teeth adjacent to the floss. It will gently slide right under the gum. There are now tools available to use which have the floss rewound for you. It is not an easy habit to learn, but once it is mastered it becomes second nature.

Dental floss is not biodegradable and should never be flushed down a toilet. The NYC Department of Environmental Protection spokesperson states "treatment plants are not designed to remove dental floss from wastewater." The Sanitation Districts of Los Angeles spokesperson states "floss can combine with other items, such as single-use wipes (like baby wipes), and form balls that can grow quite sizable and can clog sewers and pumps. Sometimes these items also combine with tree roots and grease and create huge problems for sewer systems. These materials sometimes can cause sewage spills, which threaten public health and water quality."

Not too long ago (the beginning of 2019) a study of 178 women came out possibly linking the use of certain brands of dental floss to causing heart disease and or cancer. PFAs (perfluorinated alkylate substances) in some dental floss brands is being absorbed into the blood when used. Results from the study were reported in the *Journal of Exposure Science & Environmental Epidemiology*. (PFAs are also found in nonstick cookware.) The CDC cites dental floss on a list of products that could contain PFAs. The CDC as well as the EPA do agree PFAS is "a source of potential toxic exposure for humans." Studies in people have linked PHAs to liver damage and a decreased immune response. Researchers evaluated 18 types of dental floss and the chemical components. One third contained fluorine. Testing positive for fluorine equivocates to a positive PFA.

In 1978 animal studies showed PFAS toxicity and the U.S. Environmental Protection Agency did not become aware until 2000, per Phillippe Grandjean, adjunct professor of environmental health at Harvard T.H. Chan School of Public Health. He stated that because of the delay, safe drinking water standards were inhibited. On July 31, 2018, *Environmental Health* published his editorial, which included the following: "PFAS have been linked to a range of health problems, including testicular and kidney cancers, decreased birth weight, and thyroid disease. While most companies have stopped producing two forms of PFASs -perfluorooctanoic acid (PFOA) and perfluorooctane sulfuric acid (PFOS)-the chemicals persist in drinking water systems and new forms of PFASs are raising concerns."

Dr. Ken Spaeth, chief of environmental medicine at Northwell Health New York, says, "Once they are in the body, they hang around for a few years. That's one of the concerns. It's not the kind of thing that if you get it inside of you that it's gone within a couple hours. It can hang around for quite some time. Obviously the more you're exposed, the higher the levels can be."

Toothbrushes come soft, medium and hard. Although it may seem that a hard brush makes sense to clean best, it is the exact opposite. A soft toothbrush will do the better job in removing plaque from teeth and gum surfaces. Picture a pile of mayonnaise. If you use a hard toothbrush to sweep it up, you will not do more than scratch the pile. The mayonnaise is a representation of plaque. Now, if you use a soft bristle brush, you are sweeping the mayonnaise and can remove it, as you would plaque. It is recommended to brush twice a day for two solid minutes each time. Angle the toothbrush so it is half on your teeth, and half on your gums.

You want to brush in the direction your teeth grow. Brush upward on the bottom, and downward on the top. You do not want to brush back and forth as this can be too rough on the gums, causing recession and tooth sensitivity. If you are using an electric or battery-operated toothbrush, the bristles will do the work for you. Toothbrushes should be replaced every three to four months, according to the ADA. If bristles are frayed or you are post viral infection, replacement is recommended. There are on average 2500 bristles on each toothbrush. The bristles are clumped together forming 40 tufts per brush. The Broxodent was the name of the first electric toothbrush. It was created 1954 in Switzerland and 1960 was the first electric toothbrush sale in the US. It is best to let a toothbrush dry without a cover so as not to trap bacteria.

In the Middle East, instead of giving small change, merchants sometimes give out chewing gum. Seventy-nine percent of people in the Middle East and fifty-nine percent of people in the U.S. chew gum. Chewing a mint-based flavor gum will make fruits and vegetables taste bitter. Sometimes chewing gum on one side of your mouth over the other can cause pain in the TMJ, head and or ears. Bloating is sometimes an effect of gum as the air swallowed causes the pain and bloating. This is especially noticeable in people suffering with IBS (irritable bowel syndrome). Sometimes excessive stomach acid is produced from enzymes released while chewing gum.

According to one study on amalgam fillings and gum chewing, mercury vapor when amalgams are present in the mouth, get released at a higher rate when chewing gum. Once the mercury vapor gets released, it makes its way into the bloodstream and there it will oxidize with tissues.

A study done with 30 participants between the ages of 6 and 19 looked at the relationship between gum chewing and headaches. All participants were sufferers of migraines or headaches that were chronic. After one month of no gum chewing 19 participants had zero headaches and 7 had less frequent headaches. It was believed the reduction was due to either less stress on TMJ muscles and/or the aspartame.

Artificial sweeteners found in gum have the potential to cause gastrointestinal symptoms. All gum ingredients, including aspartame, get absorbed into your body through your mouth tissue. The digestive system does not filter anything as it is bypassed. Aspartame is present in sugar-free gums as well as sugar gums. Aspartame is metabolized inside your body into both wood alcohol (a poison) and formaldehyde (which is a carcinogen used as embalming fluid and is not eliminated from your body through the normal waste filtering done by your liver and kidneys). It's been linked to birth defects, cancers, brain tumors, and weight gain. Aspartame, to reiterate, is present not only in sugar-free gums but is also present in gums containing sugar.

Sucralose (also called Splenda) is another common artificial sweetener found in gum. Only two studies were done on humans before the FDA approved this sweetener. One study, which was the longer of the two, was four days long. Animal studies of sucralose found lowered red blood cells (anemia sign), increase in mortality, and kidneys that became enlarged.

Some other questionable ingredients in chewing gum are the following. BHT is a preservative found in chewing gums and in food. A lot of other countries have banned BHT. BHT has been linked to organ system toxicity, including kidney and liver damage, hyperactivity in children, and may be carcinogenic.

Calcium casein peptone is mainly found in one popular sugar-free gum brand. The long-term studies have not been completed as of yet. Also known as calcium phosphate, this is derived from milk and highly processed.

Titanium dioxide is in gum for whitening. It's been linked to autoimmune disorders, asthma, and Crohn's disease and is potentially carcinogenic, especially in its nanoparticle form.

Plastics in our environment and food supply have become a concern. Gum is no exception to this. Most gums do contain plastic and can sometimes be disguised under the title of gum base or polyvinyl acetate. chemistry.About. com tells us that chicle (tree sap) was an original ingredient in chewing gum. Chicle, a natural rubber, got replaced after WW II with rubbers that are synthetic.

While it is important to keep your mouth clean, it is a good idea to find out what ingredients are in toothpastes or chewing gum so you can be aware of exactly what you are putting into your mouth.

CHAPTER 9
IT'S A DOG'S LIFE

Scientists believe there are almost two million species of animals in the world. Animals as well as people are attracted to smiles.

Goats were shown two photos of the same person, with only one of these photos showing that person smiling. The goats chose the smiling photo to go and explore.

Dogs are able to recognize emotions on our faces beyond just a smile. It has been shown that dogs will pick the left side of the face to look at, given the choice. And dogs can distinguish between happiness and anger, given a photo with only 25 percent of one's face being shown.

Horses can also differentiate moods on human faces. Studies have shown they will be leery of a frown and respond with positivity to someone they see smiling now, or who they have seen smiling in the past.

In order to categorize species, experts classify species into broad a classification known as genus, which are then classified into a smaller group called a family. The classification continues until the living organism can no longer be grouped further. Every classification of living organism belongs to one kingdom, of which there are five in total. These kingdoms are known as Animals, Plants, Fungi, Protista, and Monera.

Groups of monkeys are called missions, tribes, troops or carloads. Monkeys are like humans in that they each have their own set of fingerprints. They also have day and night like humans where sleeping is done primarily at night. The average sleep per day for a human is 8 hours and for a monkey is close to 10 hours. Monkeys also have two legs and two arms and are considered one of the smartest of animals. Monkeys in Thailand have been observed flossing their teeth and even teaching their children how to do so. The long-tailed macaque species of monkeys were seen using coconut fibers or twigs as floss.

Be careful if you visit because they are experienced at using human hair of the visitors as well in order to floss. Monkeys, like humans, have 16 upper and 16 lower teeth.

ANIMALS AND THEIR MOUTHS

Gray squirrels have two sets of teeth like humans and lose their primary teeth around the age of 4-5 months. They only have 6 primary teeth and, for their permanent teeth, 18 molars and 4 incisors. Every year their incisors grow approximately 6 inches. Incisors on a gray squirrel will keep erupting and run the risk of puncturing the opposite arch. This can cause the squirrel to die. Once a month captive squirrels with malocclusion need their incisors cut down and are "non-releasable" animals. The front surface of their incisors is harder than the back. White is the color seen on the back of the teeth and orange is on the front. Gray squirrels live all around the world and there are over 200 species.

Giraffes do not have upper front teeth to eat with. Since they have long tongues (18 inches) they are able to use the tongue along with their lips to grab food. The tongue is known as prehensile, meaning the tongue can be used like a hand to grab things. Thirty-two lower teeth are present in a giraffe's mouth and most are molars. Giraffes only drink a couple times a week. Their necks are not long enough to reach the ground, and have seven vertebrae just like human necks.

Cattles also do not have upper front teeth. All ruminant animals have a tough dental pad on their top lip instead of top front teeth. They have two lower canines - one on each side – which, unlike human teeth, are not pointed. By looking at the mouth of cattle one can tell how old they are. A cattle dentition is made up of six incisors, two canines, twelve premolars and twelve molars for a total of thirty-two teeth, like humans. Some calves are born with teeth and some are not. Eight primary incisors have erupted by one month of age. A "solid mouth cow" means all teeth are present. A "broken mouth cow" means some teeth are falling out.

Young and middle-aged cows are considered "solid mouth" while older cows are considered "broken mouth." Cows chew for up to 1/3 of every day at the rate of about 45 times per minute. They eat an average of 40 pounds of food daily and drink an average of 15 gallons of water daily. Only females are cows. Bulls are the males. Females (cows) are heifers until birthing a calf. George Washington's dentist made him dentures out of cow, hippopotamus and walrus teeth.

Congenital abnormalities including cleft palate, prognathic and brachhygnathia are rare, and most lesions affecting the mouth are caused by trauma and infection. Cattle with lesions of the mouth usually present with abundant salivation and weak abdominal fill due to harmed feeding. When cleft palate is drastic, calves are put to sleep.

"Wooden tongue" may be caused from hay with thistles in it. These animals are unable to eat due to a firm and protruded tongue and excessive salivating. These animals are given antibiotic treatment for approximately one week and are put in isolation.

"Lumpy jaw," also called "actinomycosis," will sometimes cause osteomyelitis in the upper cheek and lower jaw. The lower jaw will become very swollen, and sometimes the sinuses discharge. Antibiotic treatment is prescribed but the prognosis is not favorable.

Jaw fractures in cattle are mostly caused by tractor wheels hitting them. Due to pain the animals do not eat. Excessive drooling is common due to the tongue protrusion. Palpation and X-ray are two ways to determine a fracture. Antibiotic treatment may or may not be warranted. Soft foods and isolated feeding for displacements that are slight can begin healing. Displaced, open and pathological fractures necessitate emergency slaughter for welfare reasons.

Cows and horses are herbivores as they eat plants. Cows never eat meat. Pigs are omnivores as they eat meat and plants. Dogs and lions are carnivores as they eat meat. Horses, donkeys and sheep are herbivores but do not chew the cud. They are non-ruminants. Cattle, goats, sheep and buffalo chew the cud. They are ruminants.

An adult ruminant will have 32 permanent teeth after their 20 primary teeth are exfoliated.

Horses and donkeys have both primary and permanent dentitions. The brain of a horse weighs less than the teeth of a horse. In their primary set 24 teeth will be present followed by 36-44 permanent ones. Horses are born without teeth, which begin to erupt at around 2-3 weeks of age. When horses chew it is in a circular motion, and their lower jaw can be seen sliding on their top teeth. Horses' teeth do not stop growing and can last at least until around the age of 30 years, and grinding keeps teeth from growing too long. Primary teeth usually fall out between the ages of 2.5 and 5 years. Sharp edges or "hooks" can appear on a horse's teeth.

The process of filing these down is known as "floating." Hooks are caused by the sideways chewing motion of a horse. Since horses don't eat grass, which is coarse, but eat more grain products, teeth do not wear down evenly. It is recommended that horses have yearly dental checkups. The saying "long in the tooth" comes from horses. They get gum recession as they get older. The recession gives the illusion that the teeth are growing.

There are six types of sheep. Lambs are baby sheep, less than a year old. Weaners are sheep that are no longer nursing and are self-sufficient in feeding to survive. Hoggets are not at the adult stage yet but they are older than weaners. Wethers are males only and they are for the production of wool. Ewes are the female version of wethers. Rams are male adult sheep. They are for both breeding and producing wool. Sheep are like humans as they have 32 permanent teeth.

Malnutrition and weight loss happen when sheep have "broken mouth," which is when they lose incisor teeth prematurely. There is not a preventable way to stop this and it is a big issue in sheep dentition. Sheep that average 2-4 years of age sporadically show dentigerous cysts. It is not clear what causes them, so there is no way to prevent them from forming. Older sheep lose weight when the teeth are unevenly worn. This causes malocclusion and malnutrition. When eating, sheep with molar teeth problems often have pieces of fibrous feed protruding from the corners of the mouth and frequently drop large wads of masticated fibrous food from the mouth (quidding). A sheep's body condition is dependent upon a healthy dentition. A sheep known as "full mouth" has all their permanent teeth in.

Cats have more teeth in their maxillary arch than in their mandibular arch. They have 16 upper teeth and 14 lower teeth. The four canines in a cat's mouth are sharp enough to pierce through skin. The primary teeth begin to erupt in the first month of life and will all be lost by around nine months of age. There are three main mouth issues that affect cats and they are periodontal issues, resorption of teeth and stomatitis. Only 30% of cats aged 3 years are not affected by periodontal disease. One noticeable sign is bad breath. Another is plaque and or tarter above the gum line. If professional dental cleanings are not sought, plaque and tarter can turn to gingivitis. This is the red swollen gums and sometimes includes bleeding.. Gingivitis progresses into periodontitis if not addressed. Plaque bacteria below the gum line secrete toxic substances that cause further tissue damage.

These bacteria, as well as the inflammation and tissue damage they cause, often stimulate a cat's immune system. The immune system brings in white blood cells and other inflammatory chemicals to try to destroy the bacterial invaders. Periodontitis happens when the supporting tissues become damaged. A cat's premolar teeth are most commonly susceptible to a tooth root abscess. This occurs once there is active periodontal disease and the bacteria enter the roots of the cat's teeth.

Kittens do teethe but it is not for an extended period of time. Kittens will have a mouth of 30 permanent teeth by approximately 6 or 7 months of age. Their primary dentition is made up of 26 teeth which start erupting at about two weeks of age. Due to the shape of a cat's tooth, they do not get the same type dental caries like humans or even dogs. Resorption is an issue noticed in the cat mouth.

The longest canine in the animal world goes to the hippopotami. Their canines can grow to almost two feet long.

Some snail species have more than 20,000 teeth. They are located on the snail's tongue and are set in rows.

Although dolphins have teeth, their food is not chewed. There are no muscles present in a dolphin's jaw. Rings are located inside their teeth and thus the age can be determined. They do not have a second set of teeth that erupts.

Sharks lose about 4 teeth per month. They get replaced by the tooth in the row behind rather quickly.

The horns that narwhals have are actually teeth. Monodon monoceros, as they are formally called, are of Greek origin meaning "one-tooth one-horn." These horns have been known to exceed 8 feet in length.

The blue whale is the largest mammal worldwide. Krill, or tiny shrimp is all they eat so they do not need teeth and they do not have them.

Toads do not have any teeth, but frogs do.

A mosquito's teeth cannot be seen unless magnification is used. Forty-seven teeth are present in their mouth.

Abscesses that are full of white blood cells have been known to appear in a cat's mouth and are also called pus. Surgical extractions by a veterinarian are warranted, and one telltale sign is a cat will show is swelling right underneath the eye that is soft and painful. There is also a chance the tooth will fall out on its own due to mobility. In addition to local damage in the mouth, periodontal disease may also result in widespread organ damage. Organ damage from periodontal disease occurs when bacteria from the infected teeth, roots and gums gain access to the bloodstream (a condition called bacteremia). Brushing cats' teeth at home should start very early in age. Daily brushing as well as professional dental visits and cleaning by a veterinarian are the best ways to keep your cat's mouth in optimal health.

Goats have 8 incisors in their lower arch and 24 molars in this arch as well. They are edentulous (having no teeth) in their upper arch. Rather they like other animals have a "dental pad" for chewing. The first of their primary teeth, if not present at birth, erupts around one week old. And the first permanent tooth appears at around age one to one and a half years of age. Goats are thought to get their speech pattern from their environment and can pick up different accents. (Elephants can also speak with an accent from their surroundings.) Goats live on average 15-18 years. Goats are plant eaters and are equipped with special digestion to break down plant matter. They will, however, taste almost anything before deciding if it is edible. They are trainable and will know their name when you call them. Two jaw abnormalities that occur in goats are "monkey mouth" which is an "overshot jaw" and "parrot mouth" which is an "undershot jaw." Goats live as long as dogs do and have been known to bond with their owners like a dog will as well.

Dogs are known as diphyodonts, having two sets of teeth. Forty-two teeth make up the permanent dentition and 28 teeth are in a dog's primary dentition. Between three and five months is when dogs will begin to lose their primary teeth. By seven to eight months of age dogs should have all of their permanent teeth in place. A dog's dental state can affect their overall health as well. Brushing their teeth at home, in addition to professional cleanings, keeps them in optimal dental and body health. It is necessary to use general anesthesia for a proper and thorough cleaning of a canine's teeth.

DENTAL CARE FOR YOUR ANIMAL

Dental cleanings without the use of general anesthetic are available in some veterinarian offices. However, the American Animal Hospital Association (AAHA) defines anesthesia-free dentistry as "unacceptable and below the standard of care" while the American Veterinary Dental College (AVDC) has even issued a position statement warning against its use. Only twenty percent of dogs at the age of 3 years old are immune to periodontal problems. Sometimes a dental cleaning is not elective but rather a medical necessity.

Tarter accumulating underneath their gums can cause bleeding, soreness, pain and red gums. The bacteria can travel in the bloodstream and land in organs such as kidney and liver and even the heart. A dog's lifespan can be affected as chronic gum issues can put stress on organs and immunity. Pulse therapy antibiotics are considered an alternative to anesthesia for dogs that cannot undergo general anesthetic due to other health issues. In pulse therapy, antibiotics are given one week a month to the dog in order to lower the mouth bacteria amount. Sometimes after a dental cleaning with anesthesia, the dog's energy increases as the bacteria is removed, causing pain to dissipate.

The American Kennel Club Canine Health Foundation sites the following as possible complications from general anesthetic: low blood pressure, low heart rate, low blood oxygen, low body temperature, and prolonged recovery. Blood work will most likely be required prior to having this procedure(dental prophylaxis) done. Levels of kidneys and liver are checked, as well as basic blood levels. Antibiotics before the procedure may be prescribed as well. The reasons can be bacteria in the mouth at a high level, liver issues and/or heart problems. Also, dogs are now hooked up to advanced monitoring systems that track their oxygen saturation, level of exhaled carbon dioxide, blood pressure, electrical cardiac functioning and temperature, and they will beep if there are major problems, but it is equally important that a dog's heart and lung function is carefully and frequently monitored by somebody who is experienced with side effects of anesthetic drugs.

The dental cleaning, that is, scaling, polishing and x-rays, often done by veterinary technicians, but a veterinarian should always be supervising the treatment. There will most likely be IV fluids given to the dog during the dental cleaning. According to Banfield Applied Research and Knowledge, every year a dog ages comes with a 20 percent higher risk factor of having periodontal disease. They also state toy and mini dogs have a higher incidence over large breeds. The tarter that is not visible underneath the gums is the tarter that is doing the most damage.

The American Veterinary Dental College does not recommend giving cow hooves, dried natural bones or hard nylon products as these are very hard and can result in fractured teeth and damaged gums. These products do not mimic the effect of meat being pulled off a carcass as dogs would have done in the wild. Sharon Hoffman is a Diplomate of the AVDC and she also has some things to avoid giving dogs. They include soup bones, knuckle bones and some rawhide. Dr. Peter Dobias is a veterinarian who recommends no beef, buffalo, or bison shank due to the risk of teeth cracking since these bones are harder than the dog's teeth - due to the hardness of the bone. He also says that antlers cause a high number of fractures in teeth. Pork and rib bones, per Dr. Tobias, have a high risk of splintering. Dr. Karen Becker recommends not feeding dogs cooked bones due to splinter risks. Cooked bones are also void of many nutrients. The steamed and smoked bones in the stores are processed and so they too have the risk of becoming brittle. Canine teeth are the most common teeth for a dog or cat to break. Incisors are known for their wear, as dogs are rough when they chew with their front teeth.

YOUR PET'S TONGUE

There are some unique facts about dogs' tongues. Both Chow Chows and Shar-peis are Chinese breeds of dog and both have blue (or dark colored) tongues. This does make it more difficult for a veterinary diagnosis. There are over 600 bacteria types on a dog's tongue and that same number holds true for a human tongue. Dogs' tongues are smooth where a cat's tongue is covered in papillae. That makes a cat tongue better for keeping hair tangle free. Dogs have sweat glands but only on their noses and their pads on the paws. Thermoregulation is the process of cooling themselves down by panting. Macroglossia is a rare condition where a dog is born with a tongue that is too large. The sound of a dog's bark is determined by their tongue. Cats do not have as many taste buds as dogs do. And humans have more taste buds than dogs. Dogs have the ability to differentiate between bitter, salty, sweet and sour. However, cats can only taste bitter, salty and sour. Dogs have a heightened sense of smell and choose their food with this sense. Dogs and cats both use their tongues to taste water, but the process is very different.

A cat uses the tip of its tongue to pull water upward and then quickly snaps its jaw shut to catch the liquid in his mouth. A dog uses a simple lapping process with the tongue curled slightly backward to form a spoon that collects as much water as possible and quickly puts it back into their mouth. Human saliva measures around 7.0 and a dog's saliva measures about 8.5. This makes a dog's saliva more alkaline than humans. No enzymes needed for digestion are in a dog's saliva. The stomach of a dog will take care of all digestion needs. Humans do have enzymes in saliva, and digestion begins to take place as chewing takes place for humans.

WHAT TO AVOID GIVING YOUR DOG

According to caninejournal.com there are 28 foods you should never feed your dog. Water is the only safe liquid for dogs to drink. Coffee and/or tea are not safe as caffeine poisoning can happen with only a small amount of caffeine. Grapes and raisins are toxic to dogs and should never be fed to them. Kidney failure can happen from the juice of grapes. Lactose intolerance is common in adult dogs, and dairy should not be given to dogs. Apple seeds are toxic to dogs because the casing has amygdalin. When digested, this natural chemical releases cyanide. Persin is in avocados, especially in the pit. It can cause gastro problems and heart congestion. Xylitol, found in candy, gum, mouthwash and toothpaste, can cause vomiting and liver problems.

Dogs cannot digest cat food as the protein and fat levels are not suitable for dogs. In extreme cases eating cat food can cause a dog to get pancreatitis. The most dangerous chocolate for a dog to ingest is cocoa powder. No chocolate is healthy for a dog to have due to theobromine, as well as caffeine. Increased heart rate, diarrhea and in extreme amounts death can occur. Garlic and onions can be hazardous for dogs to ingest. Decreased red blood counts leading to anemia can occur. Onions in any form can damage cells in a dog. Hops, an ingredient in beer, can cause death in a dog. Human vitamin supplements are not recommended for dogs.

The worst culprit is prenatal vitamins which can be toxic, due to the increased iron. Macadamia nuts are not safe for dogs, not even in tiny amounts. Rhubarb and tomato leaves both have oxalates which are not safe for dogs. Sodium ion poisoning can happen when dogs have too much salt. Any type of sugar runs the risk of diabetes and dental issues. Tobacco poisoning can show up in as little as one hour in a dog. Too much yeast can expand a dog's stomach so much that it ruptures. There is some conflicting information on a few of these items, but for the most part it is the same.

CHAPTER 10
BUT WAIT THERE'S MORE

FUN FACTS

Brad Pitt had his front tooth chipped on purpose when he played Tyler Durden in "Fight Club."

Wisdom teeth are named "love teeth" in Korea.

"Bluetooth" comes from King Harold Blatand (Danish) because his teeth stained blue. This was because he ate so many blueberries.

Simple assault in Louisiana is when natural teeth are used to bite someone.

Aggravated assault in Louisiana is when false teeth are used to bite someone.

Cats need taurine to keep fur, teeth and eyesight intact.

When Ben Affleck filmed "Armageddon" he underwent approximately $20,000 of cosmetic dentistry. He built out and whitened his small sized teeth, which were not spaced uniformly, at the request of the director.

In Japan "Yaeba" is the name given to non-perfect teeth. It is looked upon as a positive characteristic.

Roald Dahl, author of *Charlie and the Chocolate Factory*, had a full mouth of extractions at age 21. He didn't want to be bothered taking care of them.

Wisdom teeth contain stem cells.

It is mandatory to have all of your wisdom teeth extracted and your appendix removed in order to work in Antarctica.

Jim Carrey has a chipped front tooth, as seen in "Dumb and Dumber."

Every year over five million teeth are knocked out.

Knocked out teeth can be saved by placing them back in the socket quickly or by saving in a glass of milk. Be careful not to touch the roots.

Over one hundred billion dollars per year is spent on dental care in America.

Soft toothbrushes are recommended by dental professionals as the bristles sweep away bacteria.

Hard toothbrushes are not recommended as they scratch tooth surfaces.

About one quarter of adults do not brush twice daily.

About twenty five percent of adults are edentulous (toothless).

Three hundred types of bacteria are in your mouth, at least.

Over fourteen million gallons of toothpaste are sold in America yearly.

Barbers as well as blacksmiths practiced dentistry in the 1800s.

Taste buds have a ten-day life span.

Approximately twenty-five hundred bristles are in each toothbrush.

There are no muscles in a dolphin's jaw so their teeth do not chew, they only grab.

In your lifetime you average 38 1/2 days brushing your teeth.

Children miss 51 million hours of school each year due to dental issues.

Lucy Beaman was the first licensed female dentist (1866).

In 1905 Irene Newman became the first dental hygienist.

A common wedding gift in the British Isles was dentures.

95% of adult diabetics have periodontal disease.

The average American spends 48 seconds brushing their teeth.

Cavities are more common than asthma.

You tend to chew food on the same side you write with.

The first toothbrush was made from twigs.

There is a crocodile bird which cleans the crocodile's teeth. The bird flies into the open mouth of the crocodile.

The definition of odontalgia is toothache.

In 1728 the first braces were made (France).

Dental floss was first manufactured in 1882.

Dogs have 42 teeth.

Cats have 30 teeth.

Blue whales have 0 teeth.

There are no premolars in a set of baby teeth.

There are 32 teeth in permanent dentition if you include wisdom teeth.

Jaw size decreased as brain size increased.

Enamel is 96% hydroxyapatite.

Primary teeth are whiter than permanent teeth.

People prefer blue toothbrushes over red ones.

Craze lines are the cracks you see in your front teeth and are normal.

Clefts are sometimes seen in dogs, but rarely in cats.

The average amount of money the tooth fairy left in 1950 was 25 cents.

Perez the mouse (Ratoncito Perez) is the Spanish tooth fairy (Madrid 1894).

A mouse has teeth that never stop growing.

Saliva is 99 percent water and 1 percent electrolytes and organic substances.

Your bite can cause your shoe heels to wear unevenly.

In the Middle Ages kissing a donkey was a custom if you had a toothache.

The hardest surface in your body is the enamel on your teeth.

Teeth are not bones as they cannot regenerate themselves.

100,000 gallons of saliva are produced on average in each American's lifetime.

The first bristle toothbrush was made in China in 1498.

Cheese can protect enamel from decay.

Your tongue print is like your fingerprint - one of a kind.

The most choked on item in America is a toothpick.

When a sore jaw is accompanied with chest pain, it can mean a heart attack.

On average, $500,000 is spent on gum every year in America.

The most popular day for dental appointments is Tuesday.

The most popular month for dental appointments is January.

A very common dream is one of losing your teeth.

Toilet flush can spray bacteria six feet, so keep your toothbrush at least that far away.

The only muscle to be attached just by one side is the tongue.

The weakest of the five senses is taste.

Only 15 percent of people cannot roll their tongue.

Clenching your left thumb into your left fist stops you from gagging.

Wait to brush after eating or drinking acidic products.

Giraffes only have lower teeth.

In Vermont it is not legal for a woman to wear false teeth, unless they have written permission of their husband.

There is such a thing as a tooth tattoo.

Your teeth are alive.

Teeth have been used in witchcraft spells.

Use dental floss to cut a cake perfectly.

Dental floss can be used to start a fire.

Dental floss can double as thread.

Cells in urine have been used in China to grow teeth.

Two thirds of your teeth are not above the gum line.

Toothpaste can clean scuffed shoes.

Toothpaste can be used to clean piano keys.

It is actually the posture of your tongue that determines whether or not you look attractive to others.

DDS and DMD are both dentists with the same education. The initials differ depending on the school attended. The degree received is determined by the university and both DDS and DMD receive the same curriculum and training.

A prosthodontist specializes in crown and bridge work.

Crest toothpaste added fluoride in 1955 and was first to do so.

The pineal gland (your third eye) is where fluoride calcifies.

Listerine was once distilled and marketed as a floor cleaner.

BPA can form once saliva comes in contact with a dental filling.

"You don't know what you don't know. But hopefully now there is a little less that you don't know."

"When you change the way you look at things, the things you look at will change."

Please visit Cindy Grossmann's websites,
Dentistryshakenandstirred.com
Brilliantsmilesbycindy.com

You can also connect with her:
Email - Cindy@brilliantsmilesbycindy.com
Facebook - Cindy May Grossmann
Instagram - Cindy.m.Grossmann
LinkedIn - Cindy Grossmann

www.ingramcontent.com/pod-product-compliance
Lightning Source LLC
Chambersburg PA
CBHW060839220526
45466CB00003B/1164